SCIENCE OF HEALING

A Comprehensive Commentary on the Root Tantra and
Diagnostic Techniques of Tibetan Medicine

by

Dr. Tenzing Dakpa

DORRANCE PUBLISHING CO., INC.
PITTSBURGH, PENNSYLVANIA 15222

To my mentors, Doctors Yeshi Dhonden and Tenzin Choedrak, the former and late senior personal physicians to His Holiness the XIV Dalai Lama, for their limitless instructions and kindness during the years I spent with them.

This book recounts the experiences of a single individual and is not meant to serve the reader or anyone else as medical advice. Please consult your physician before beginning any program of physical or mental health treatment.

ISBN: 978-0-8059-7432-4
Library of Congress Control Number: 2006930388

Printed in the United States of America

First Printing

For more information or to order additional books, please contact:
Dorrance Publishing Co., Inc.
701 Smithfield Street
Third Floor
Pittsburgh, Pennsylvania 15222
U.S.A.
1-800-788-7654
www.dorrancebookstore.com

CONTENTS

Examining the Characteristics of a Nasal Disorder
Examining the Tongue
    Examining the Characteristics of a Tongue Disorder
Examining the Lips
    Examining the Characteristics of a Lip Disorder
Examining the Complexion
Examining the Sputum
Examining the Feces
Examining the Vomiting
Examining the Blood
    The Characteristics of Unhealthy Blood
    The Characteristics of Healthy Blood

Finding the Causative Factors of an Illness
Finding the Sites of an Illness
Finding the Signs and Symptoms

    Abstract
    BDORT and Professor Omura
    O-Ring Test Life Science Research Institute and Shimotsuura Hospital
    The Preceding Conditions about the Patients' Case Presentation
    Actual Case Presentation

List of Tables

List of Illustrations

PREFACE

As a Tibetan, I love my country and fellow countrymen. I have great respect for the rich cultural heritage for which Tibet is known all over the world. My connection with traditional Tibetan medicine began in Dharamsala, India, the seat of Tibetan Government in Exile, in the summer of 1981. Here, I worked as an assistant-cum-translator to Dr. Yeshi Dhonden, the former personal physician to H. H. the XIVth Dalai Lama of Tibet for six years. I often sat opposite Dr. Dhonden during his working hours in his consulting room. He sees patients of all faiths and nationalities. They come to see him from distant places like Chandigarh, Delhi, and Bombay with great faith and respect. I paid great attention to his practice and admired his patience, diligence, and service.

Dr. Dhonden is my uncle from the maternal side and was also my first teacher of Tibetan medicine. I learned many things from him and have great respect for his service to Tibetan medicine. Dr. Tashi Yarphel Tashigang and his wife, Dawa-la, old and close friends of Dr. Dhonden, often came to Dharamsala from Delhi. They gave me many books on Tibetan medicine and always encouraged me to pursue its study. I greatly value their advice and kindness. From time to time, Venerable Lhundup Yeshe-la, another uncle from my maternal side, reminded me to put more effort into learning Tibetan medicine. I regard his kindness and straightforward advice highly.

The friendship and guidance of Patricia (Trisha) Walsh changed my direction. She often came to Dr. Dhonden for practical training during working hours and in the evenings for medical teachings. It was through her that I learned of the two Medicine Buddha Empowerments I received from Kyabje Dilgo Khyentse Rinpoche (head of the Nyingma School of Tibetan Buddhism) at Men-Tsee-Khang (the Tibetan Medical and Astrological Institute of H. H. the XIVth Dalai Lama). It was also through her that I learned that Men-Tsee-Khang was seeking new students. I enrolled in March of 1987. Her guidance was instrumental for who I am today and I therefore regard her friendship of great value.

At Men-Tsee-Khang I received medical teachings from Professors Lobsang Choephel, Pasang Yonten Arya, Tenpa Choephel Tepel, and Lobsang Tenzin Rinpoche. I received basic teachings on Tibetan Elemental Astrology from Professor Drakton Jampa Gyaltsen and further teachings on grammar and the basics of Buddhist philosophy from Professor Dorjee Gyalpo. I received further training on the identification of medicinal plants from Professors (Bu) Dawa, Lobsang Tenzin Rinpoche, and Tenpa Choephel Tepel.

I graduated from Men-Tsee-Khang College at the top of its seventh batch of students. I then received my practical training under Dr. Kunga Gyurmey Nyarongsha (the late personal physician to H. H. the XIVth Dalai Lama) at the Nizamuddin branch clinic in New Delhi, India. I learned many things from accompanying Dr. Lobsang Wangyal (the late personal physician to H. H. the XIVth Dalai Lama) as his assistant-cum-translator to Kolkata (Calcutta), Bhubaneshwar, and Bangalore.

I also learned many things as a special assistant to Dr. Tenzin Choedrak (the late senior personal physician to H. H. the XIVth Dalai Lama) in Dharamsala for seven years from 1995 to 2001. I accompanied Dr. Choedrak to Delhi, Tabo, and Chennai in India as well as to Europe, the United States, and Canada. He loved his practice and was humble and very compassionate to all the patients. He always received his patients with great care and love and made no distinction between rich or poor. He was knowledgeable, experienced, and had great affection for Men-Tsee-Khang.

During his tenure as thirteenth director of Men-Tsee-Khang from 1995 to 1998, Tsering Tashi Phuri worked very hard in promoting Tibetan medicine and astrology as well as in improving the overall working standards of administration, various departments, staff, and students. He always came early in the morning and stayed late in the evening to keep his office job up to date. During the day, he visited different departments to inspect the work he assigned to the staff and the departments. He also called meetings from time to time to discuss the development and direct the course of the administration. He was very good in overseeing administration jobs and making connections with other organizations. Under his directorship, Men-Tsee-Khang developed tremendously. Men-Tsee-Khang misses his directorship and he is admired by most of the staff. In my opinion, he is the most outstanding director Men-Tsee-Khang has had so far.

The seed for this book was actually sown during the early eighties while I was working under Dr. Yeshi Dhonden. However, it took many long years to complete due to lack of facilities and reference books. The main inspiration for completing this book came from traditional Tibetan doctors in Tibet and in exile. Doctors Yeshi Dhonden and Tenzin Choedrak's tireless work to advance this science was particularly inspirational.

Though it is just a drop, my intention is to elucidate the vast treasures of *rGyud.bZhi* (the Four Tantras), on which I have spent so many years, seeking to understand and unearth its profound meaning. I have tried to back up the main topics with relevant information and notes from many references. For instance, though the said seat of *Rlung Thur.Sel* (Downward Voiding *Rlung*) is the anal canal, I think it is the sacral region. My belief is based on the understanding I have gained from reading, studying, and researching the functions of the nervous system. It is also supported by a line from the eighty-sixth chapter of the Oral Instruction's Tantra on wounds of the extremities, which says that the central and peripheral nervous systems function because of *Rlung* moving in them.

I have tried to present the most comprehensive guide to diagnosis by pulse and urine examination ever to appear in English. I have tried to clarify many critical points of pulse and urine examination. I have also included a guide to the twelve subjects of secondary examination, including personality and appearance of eyes and interrogation. Finally comes "Tibetan Medicine and the BDORT" (Bi-Digital O-Ring Test), a talk I gave at the Sixteenth International Symposium on Acupuncture and Electro-Therapeutics at Columbia University, New York City in 2000. The International College of Acupuncture and Electro-Therapeutics and The New York Academy of Medicine holds a symposium every year at the above venue.

This talk contains the case histories of twelve patients I saw with my colleague, Dr. Dawa, at the O-Ring Test Life Science Research Institute and Shimotsuura Clinic in Kurume, Fukuoka, Japan in 2000. Professor Yasuhiro Shimotsuura and his associates at the above clinic arranged the patients' consultation as well as provided their medical reports from their respective files to confirm my findings. I also received immense assistance from Shigeharu Fukuda Ph.D. and Takashi Shibuya during my preparation for this talk. However, without the kindness and financial support of Mr. Ken Hayashibara, the President of the Hayashibara Biochemical Laboratory in Okayama, Japan, nothing would have materialized. He is a strong supporter of Tibetan medicine and Tibetan culture. I have high esteem for his kindness and support.

As explained by Professor Yoshiaki Omura during his three-day workshop at the Men-Tsee-Khang hall in the summer of 1999, BDORT is a simple, non-invasive, safe, and quick new diagnostic method developed by him in the early 1970s. According to Professor Omura, physicians in the U.S.A., Scandinavian countries, Germany, Belgium, England, Japan, China, Korea, and Venezuela have been using this technique since the early 1980s. He made the statement: "Tibetan medicine is the most advanced medicine in the world before the development of modern western medical science. In combination with the BDORT, Tibetan medicine can become a very powerful too!" He is an adjunct professor of preventive medicine at New York Medical College; professor of Non-Orthodox Medicine of Ukrainian National Medical University, Kiev, Ukraine; director of the Heart Disease Research Foundation, and the president of the International College of Acupuncture & Electro-Therapeutics, based in New York, U.S.A.

I have used the Wylie system to transliterate the names of Tibetan books and medical terms. Base characters are indicated with a capital letter and syllables are separated by a period.

I am extremely indebted to Men-Tsee-Khang for my medical education and hence have great affection for it. I am wishing a mom-like Men-Tsee-Khang success in accomplishing its goal of reaching out to all.

Finally, I take full responsibility for any errors in the material. It is my sincere desire that this work may contribute to the unearthing of the treasures of the Science of Healing.

ACKNOWLEDGMENTS

I pay homage to the three ancestral Dharma Kings: Songtsen Gampo, Trisong Deutsen, and Tri Ralpa Chen, for introducing, establishing, and supporting the Buddha Dharma and *gSo.Ba Rig.Pa* (Science of Healing) in Tibet.

Next, I pay homage to Guru Padmasambhava (the Second Buddha), the great Indian Pandits (masters), the Tibetan Lotsawas (translators), master physician Yuthog Yonten Gonpo, and other scholars for translating the Buddha Dharma and *gSo.Ba Rig.Pa* (Science of Healing) into the Tibetan language.

Finally, I pay homage to His Holiness the XIVth Dalai Lama for his supreme leadership and for securing the rich cultural heritage of Tibet by re-establishing the monasteries, institutes, and schools in exile in India. Under his auspices, Tibetans successfully preserved, promoted, and transmitted their cultures to the younger generations. I want to thank the government and people from all over the world, and particularly the host, India, for their genuine help and support in withstanding the most difficult period for Tibet. I consider their kindness and help of great value.

I am indebted to all my teachers, from elementary school to the Tibetan Medical College, for their guidance and kindness. They planted the seed that lit the lamp of knowledge of the *gSo.Ba Rig.Pa* (Science of Healing) in my heart.

I thank Professors Lobsang Tenzin Rinpoche, Menrampa Tenpa Choephel Tepel, Namgyal Qusar, Tenzin Deche Kartsang, Lobsang Dhondup, Dawa, and Tsering Dhondup for their encouragement and support.

I also thank Maurice Salen (my elder brother); Dr. Ute Vogt; Ruthie DePaul; Hue Phan and his family members; Helge Skibeli and Clora Kelly; Professor Steven Emmet, M.D. and Yuki Emmet; professor Robert A. F. Thurman and Nena Thurman of Tibet House U.S., and Professor B. Alan Wallace of Santa Barbara Institute for Consciousness Studies—for their friendship and support.

I also thank Doctors Rinzin Choedon, Tashi Yarphel Tashigang, and the Ven. Tulku Pema Wangyal Rinpoche brothers; Lhundup Yeshe; Professor Jonathan Mark Kenoyer; William Calkins, M.D.; Barbara Neebel Meier; Marsha Woolf; Susan Ahrens Arendt; and Dylan Oliver for their help and support.

I would also like to thank Duane Nelson and Marion Nelson of the Medicine Buddha Healing Center in Spring Green, Wisconsin, for their encouragement and support during my work as well as Kathy Madigan and Jill Madigan for their help in editing my work with great care and enthusiasm.

I wish to thank Shigeharu Fukuda, Ph.D., Takashi Shibuya, and Naoya Masaki of the Amase Institute; Kazuya Masaki and Mohammad Raees of the Hayashibara Biochemical Laboratory and their associates in Okayama, Japan; and Ama la Imtraut Wager and my Men-Tsee-Khang medical college sponsor, Inge Stempel, of Germany, for their immense support and kind hearts.

I also wish to thank Professor Yoshiaki Omura for his immense support and kindness; Professor Yasuhiro Shimotsuura, for granting permission to use the patients' medical reports and pictures, as well as his wife (Mrs. Yasuko Shimotsuura); and associates and the patients for their good hearts and wonderful humour.

My thanks also to my parents, Gyatso and Tsering Pelzom; sisters, Ngodup Dolma and Samten; daughters, Tenzin Phagdol, Tenzin Tsomo, Tenzin Norzin, and Tenzin Pema; and wife, Kalsang, for their encouragement, affection, and limitless kindness.

My deepest heartfelt thanks are due to Doctors Yeshi Dhonden and the late Tenzin Choedrak and Lobsang Wangyal; Patricia (Trisha) Walsh; Tsering Tashi Phuri, the president of the Tibet Center, Chicago; and Ken Hayashibara, the president of the Hayashibara Biochemical Laboratory, Okayama, Japan, for their unlimited kindness and compassion.

Dr. Tenzing Dakpa

TRANSLITERATION

I have used the Wylie transliteration system in this work since it is the simplest method for transliterating Tibetan. The following chart illustrates the Wylie transliteration system for the base letters and four vowels.

; -	Ka	D -	Kha	G -	Ga	P -	Nga
T -	Ca	V -	Cha	W -	Ja	Z -	Nya
b -	Ta	f -	Tha	h -	Da	m -	Na
q -	Pa	w -	Pha	z -	Ba	-	Ma
® -	Tsa	± -	Tsha	². -	Dza	¶ -	Wa
Ÿ -	Zha	ˌ -	Za	° -	'a	» -	Ya
1/4 -	Ra	3/4 -	La	Á -	Sha	Å -	Sa
		È -	Ha	Í -	A		
ÍÛ -	I	Í_ -	U	Íï -	E	Íô -	O

xvii

INTRODUCTION

The Tibetan medical system is one of the world's oldest known medical traditions. It is also one of the five major fields of study in Tibetan scholarship, along with the arts and crafts, grammar, logic, and philosophy. It is called *gSo.Ba Rig.Pa* (Skt: *Cikitsa Vidya*; Eng: Science of Healing) in the *rGyud.bZhi* (Four Tantras), the main medical text all Tibetan doctors study. The foundation of Tibetan medicine, on which the other systems of medicine were later incorporated, is believed to be as old as civilization itself.

The Tibetan terms for medicine and disease are *sMan* and *Nad*, respectively. The word *sMan* means to heal disease and to benefit the body, whereas *Nad* means disharmony, harm, and suffering to both the body and mind. Therefore, he or she who practices *sMan* and heals *Nad* is called a *sMan.Pa.*

Both the medical history and historians suggest that some form of medicinal practices existed during the pre-Buddhist era; however, its greatest period of development seems to have come with the advent of Buddhism from India. The first physicians to visit central Tibet from India were Biji Gaje and Bilha Gaje. They came from Bodh Gaya (Vajrasana) during the reign of the twenty-eighth king, Lha Thotho Ri Nyentsen (AD 348-468).

Later, during the reign of the thirty-third king, Songtsen Gampo (AD 617-650), Galenos[1] from Persia, Han Wang Hang De from China and Bhardwaj from India came to Tibet. With the king's encouragement, they translated their systems of medicine into Tibetan. These three systems were known as the three great medical traditions.

In the eighth century, King Trisong Deutsen (AD 718-785) convened the First International Medical Conference at Samye. Eminent physicians from India, China, Persia, East Turkestan, Mongolia, and Nepal attended this conference. Elder Yuthog Yonten Gonpo (AD 708-833) was twenty years old when he participated in this conference. It is most likely that after his third visit to India, at the age of thirty-eight, he synthesized the best of the then-known medical systems into the *rGyud.bZhi*. In it Yuthog also incorporated the medical works of Guru Padmasambhava's Nectar Essence (Tib: *bDud.rTsi sNying.Po*).

The widespread transmission and practice of *rGyud.bZhi* appears to have begun in AD 763 after the establishment of the first major medical school, called *lTa.Na.sDug*, by Yuthog at Kongpo Menlung in Southern Tibet. (See Figure 1.1 for Elder Yuthog Yonten Gonpo.) The present version of *rGyud.bZhi* was perhaps redacted by his most famous descendent, the Younger Yuthog Yonten Gonpo (AD 1126-1202).

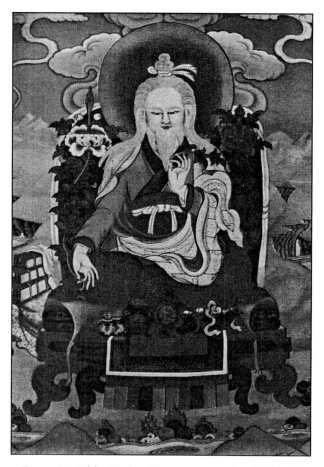

Figure 1.1: Elder Yuthog Yonten Gonpo (AD 708-833)
The Father of Tibetan Medicine and Second Medicine Buddha

This unique system of medicine is a blend of science, art, and philosophy. It is a science because its principles are enumerated in a systematic and logical framework based on an understanding of the body and its relationship to the environment. It is an art because it uses diagnostic techniques based on the creativity, insight, subtlety, and compassion of the medical practitioner. And it is a philosophy because it builds on the key Buddhist principles of altruism, karma, and ethics.

Since body and mind are seen as composites of a whole, the approach of *gSo.Ba Rig.Pa* in providing health care is holistic and non-invasive. For centuries, this has also been practiced in Bhutan, Mongolia, Buryatia (a Republic of Russia), and in the Himalayan regions of Nepal and India.

Presently, Tibetan medicine is taught at traditional Tibetan medical universities including Men-Tsee-Khang (Tibetan Medical and Astrological Institute) in Lhasa, Tibet; at the Central Institute of Higher Tibetan Studies in Sarnath; at Chagpori Medical College in Darjeeling; and at Men-Tsee-Khang in Dharamsala, India.

In exile, His Holiness the XIVth Dalai Lama re-established Men-Tsee-Khang on March 23, 1961. He appointed Dr. Yeshi Dhonden and Venerable Lodoe Gyatso as the heads of the medical and astrological sections, respectively. Initialy, Men-Tsee-Khang lacked finance, staff, and necessary facilities. At present, the head office of Men-Tsee-Khang in Dharamsala oversees the operation of various departments in Dharamsala and forty-seven branch clinics in India including four in Nepal.

The NSTG (Dutch foundation for Tibetan medicine) in Amsterdam, Netherlands, was established in September 1996. Men-Tsee-Khang in Dharamsala, India, then deputed Dr. Tenzin Deche Kartsang as its first RTHA (Resident Tibetan Health Advisor). Dr. Kartsang practiced at the above center for three years and is currently one of the three chief medical officers of the Nizamuddin branch clinic in New Delhi, India.

The Medicine Buddha Healing Center at the Global View in Spring Green, Wisconsin, U.S.A., was established in 2002 with the help of Duane Nelson and Marion Nelson. The late Doctors Tenzin Choedrak and Lobsang Wangyal had both visited this place in the 1990s. Dr. Tenzing Dakpa served at this center from May 2002 to October 2004 as its RTHA.

The work of Men-Tsee-Khang has increased over the years with the creation of the Pharmaceutical, Astrological, College, Research and Development, Materia Medica, Documentation and Publication, and the Herbal Product Research Departments, library, and museum. Men-Tsee-Khang Exports is based in New Delhi and distributes Men-Tsee-Khang products internationally.

The Men-Tsee-Khang College in Dharamsala, India, trains the Tibetan and non-Tibetan students in traditional Tibetan medicine and astrology. The course is five years long and the internship one year. The astrological department produces a range of annual almanacs, calendars, and horoscopes as well as date and times for different religious ceremonies.

Most of the herbal supplements produced by Men-Tsee-Khang go to Indians and foreigners. They have proved successful for asthma, arthritis, cardiovascular disorders including high blood pressure, gastrointestinal disorders, stress and anxiety, and a wide range of chronic illnesses. The doctors and astrologers regularly visit abroad and many places in India for conferences, seminars, consultations, and exhibitions.

Its mission is to preserve, promote, and transmit the knowledge and practice of traditional Tibetan medicine and astrology to the younger generations and to provide accessible health care to all in the twenty-first century.

Part One
The Root Tantra

CHAPTER ONE

BASIS OF DISCUSSION

The title of this work in Sanskrit is *"Amrta Hrdya Anga Ashta Guhaya Upadesha Tantra.¹"* The Tibetan title is *"bDud.rTsi sNying.Po Yan.Lag brGyad.Pa gSang.Ba Man.Ngag Gi rGyud.²"* The English title is "The Secret Oral Instructions Tantra on the Eight Branches of the Essence of Nectar."

The translation of the title follows with Tibetan, Sanskrit, and English in Table 1.1.1.

Table 1.1.1: The Title in Tibetan, Sanskrit and English

Tibetan	Sanskrit	English
bDud.rTsi	Amrta	Nectar
sNying.Po	Hrdya³	Essence
Yan.Lag	Anga	Branches
brGyad.Pa	Ashta	Eight
gSang.Ba	Guhaya	Secret
Man.Ngag Gi	Upadesha	Oral Instruction's
rGyud	Tantra	Tantra

The explanation of the title in Tibetan follows in order:

bDud.rTsi: In general, *bDud* means devil and *rTsi* means mucilaginous. The *Amrta* is a Sanskrit word, which means A (not) and *mrta* (death). The combined word *Amrta* means deathless or immortal. More often, it is translated as "nectar." The root text as well, as a commentary on synonyms called "Treasure of Immortality" (Skt: *Amarkosha*; Tib: *'Chi.Med mDzod*) explains that he who drinks nectar is immortal. But *bDud* here refers to illness and *rTsi* to medicine. Like a devil, the illness causes unrest to both body and mind. Like mucilage, the medicine

3

heals illnesses and comforts both body and mind.

sNying.Po: It's like the extraction of butter from milk. The Science of Healing is like a nectar and essence because it is extracted from many oriental medical systems. Therefore, it is also called bDud.rTsi sNying.Po (Essence of Nectar) because of its outstanding features among all medical treatises.

Yan.Lag
brGyad.Pa: Applied to trees, the Sanskrit term *Anga* means *branch*. Applied to bodies, it means *limb*. The eight limbs or branches[4] are actually the objects healed by Tibetan medicines. As ordered in the Tibetan system, these are:

(1) *Lus*[5]:   The body
(2) *Byis.Pa*:   Pediatrics
(3) *Mo.Nad*:   Gynecology
(4) *gDon*:   Disorders caused by evil spirits[6]
(5) *mTshon*:   Wounds inflicted by weapons
(6) *Dug*:   Toxicology
(7) *rGas*:   Geriatrics
(8) *Ro.Tsa*:   Aphrodisiacs

gSang.Ba: This refers to a matter which should be kept secret from certain people. It should not be taught to those suffering the three faults of a pot. The three faults are:
(1) Upside-down Pot: Fault of not paying attention to the teachings;
(2) Leaky Pot: Fault of not retaining the teachings in one's mind; and
(3) Dirty Pot: Fault of having a deluded mind.

Man.Ngag
Gi: A teacher should monitor a student's development carefully, giving further instruction only as the disciple is ready to receive it. Training should be very clear, thorough, and steady and should be transmitted both orally and through actual practice.

rGyud: The Sanskrit term *Tantra* is a combination of two words, the *Tan* (body) and *tra* (protection). It also indicates the unbroken transmission of knowledge on how to protect the body. Because the medical teachings have been transmitted from master to disciple in an unbroken lineage, it is called *rGyud*.

The homage in Tibetan is:"*bCom.lDan 'Das De.bZhin gShegs.Pa dGra bCom.Pa Yang Dag.Par rDzogs.Pa'i Sangs.rGyas sMan.Gyi Bla Vaidurya*[7] *'Od.Kyi rGyal.Po La Phyag 'Tshal.Lo*"[8]

The English translation is: "(I) prostrate to the Victorious Conqueror, Thus Gone Beyond, the Foe Destroyer, the perfectly accomplished Awakened One, Master of Medicine, and King of Vaidurya Light." The translation of the first homage follows with Tibetan, Sanskrit, and English in Table 1.1.2.

Table 1.1.2: The Homage

Tibetan	**Sanskrit**	**English**
bCom.lDan 'Das	Bhagavan	The Victorious Conqueror
De.bZhin gShegs.Pa	Tathagata	Thus Gone Beyond
dGra bCom.Pa	Arhat	Foe Destroyer
Yang Dag.Par rDzogs.Pa'i	Samayak Sam	Perfectly accomplished
Sangs.rGyas	Buddha	Awakened One
sMan.Gyi *Bla*	Baishajya Guru	Master of Medicine
Vaidurya	Vaidurya	Vaidurya
'Od.Kyi rGyal.Po (La)	Prabha Rajaya	(to) King of Light
Phyag 'Tshal.Lo	Namo	(I) prostrate

The explanation of the above Tibetan words follows in order:

bCom.lDan 'Das:	*bCom* means to conquer the four devils or evil forces of aggregates, afflictions, death, and the Son of God (*Lust*). *lDan* means the endowment of six excellent qualities,[9] and *'Das* means to transcend the realm of cyclic existence (Skt: *Samsara*; Tib: *'Khor.Ba*).
De.bZhin gShegs.Pa:	Has gone beyond cyclic existence or reached the state of omniscience by following the way of his predecessor.
dGra bCom.Pa:	Has destroyed (subdued) his inner foe, the delusive obscurations (Skt: *Klesha*; Tib: *Nyon.Mongs.Pa*) which cause suffering.

Yang Dag.Par rDzogs.Pa'i:	Has perfectly accomplished (endowed) the 112 marks of a Buddha.
Sangs.rGyas:	Has completely purified (himself) of all faults and delusions and perfected all knowledge and wisdom.
sMan.Gyi Bla:	Master of Medicine, who is supreme among the physicians.
Vaidurya:	The color of the Medicine Buddha's body is sky-like blue Vaidurya; it is very clear, transparent, and radiant.
'Od.Kyi rGyal.Po (La):	The lights radiating from the Medicine Buddha are not only brighter than the Sun's rays, but they also pacify the three mental poisons[10] and associated imbalances of *Rlung, mKhris.Pa*, and *Bad.Kan*.
Phyag 'Tshal.Lo:	Prostration signifies respect, and by doing so one also receives blessings for the successful completion of work.

The Second Homage

The homage in Tibetan is:

Thugs.rJes 'Gro.Ba'i Don.mDzad bCom.lDan 'Das
mTshan.Tsam Thos.Pas Ngan.'Gro'i sDug.bsNgal sKyob
Dug.gSum Nad.Sel Sangs.rGyas sMan.Gyi Bla
Vaidurya.Yi 'Od.La Phyag 'Tshal.Lo[11]

The English Translation is:

Out of compassion, the Victorious Conqueror benefits sentient beings
By merely hearing his name, the beings in the unfortunate realm are protected from their suffering
Master of Medicine, Awakened One, who dispels the three poisons and three disorders
To you, the Light of Vaidurya, I prostrate.

The Five Excellences

"Thus I have spoken at one time" here denotes the five excellences.[12] The translation of the five excellences follows with Tibetan, Sanskrit, and English in Table 1.1.3.

6

Table 1.1.3: The Five Excellences

Tibetan	Sanskrit	English	Connotation
'Di.sKad	Dharma sampanna	Thus	Excellent teaching
bDag.Gis	Sastra sampanna	I have	Excellent teacher
bShad.Pa'i	Parishad sampanna	Spoken	Excellent retinue
Dus.gCig	Kala sampanna	One time	Excellent period
Na	Sthana sampanna	At	Excellent abode

These are the five excellences in short form. However, some commentary is required to understand them. This elaboration follows.

Excellent Abode

In a City of Medicine called Beautiful to behold (Skt: *Sudarshana*; Tib: *lTa.Na.sDug*[13]), the abode of sages, there is a palace built from five precious human jewels.[14] This palace is adorned with various types of precious medicinal jewels that eliminate the 404 disorders[15] arising from *Rlung, mKhris.Pa, Bad.Kan*, and from dual combinations or *tri-Nyes.Pa* imbalances. They also cool hot disorders, warm cold disorders, pacify the 1,080 types of obstacles,[16] and fulfill all needs and desires.

Because of differences in their accumulation of merit and wisdom, humans, gods, and Bodhisattvas perceive the same jewels differently. As explained by Arya Nagarjuna, founder of the middle way (Madhyamaka) school of Buddhist philosophy, the qualities seen by these three classes of beings are:

The Jewels of Humans
(1) Endowed with all purifying color
(2) Pacifies harm from poison
(3) Pacifies harm from evil spirits
(4) Dispels darkness
(5) Alleviates swelling
(6) Alleviates hot disorders, etc., sufferings
(7) Fulfills wishes

The Jewels of Gods
For gods, the jewels have the former qualities and four more:
(8) Follows them everywhere
(9) Perfectly pure
(10) Have the ability to communicate
(11) Light in weight

The Jewels of Bodhisattvas
Bodhisattvas perceive the preceding eleven qualities and three more:
(12) Enable them to foresee the death and rebirth of each sentient being
(13) Enable them to foresee the time of the ultimate liberation
(14) Teachings are delivered according to the needs of all sentient beings simultaneously

To the four directions of that city lay four mountains. They are Piercing One, Snow Clad, Fragrant, and Garlanded. The explanation about these four mountains follows in order.

Piercing One Mountain
To the south of that city, there is a mountain called Piercing One (Skt: *Vindhya*; Tib: *'Bigs.Byed*), which is endowed with the power of the Sun. In this medicinal forest grows pomegranate (*Se.'Bru*), black pepper (*Na.Le.Sham*), long pepper (*Pi.Pi.Ling*), and Plumbago zeylanica (*Tsi.Tra.Ka*), which tastes hot, sour, and salty[17] with hot and sharp powers and eliminates cold disorder. The roots, trunks, branches, leaves, flowers, and fruits[18] of these medicines are fragrant, attractive, and pleasing to behold, and cold disorders do not arise wherever their scent pervades.

Snow Clad Mountain
To the north of that city, there is a mountain called Snow Clad (Skt: *Himavata*; Tib: *Gangs.Can*), which is endowed with the power of the Moon. In this medicinal forest grows sandalwood (*Tsan.Dan*), camphor (*Ga.Bur*), eaglewood (*A.Ga.Ru*), and margosa (*Nim.Pa*),[19] which tastes bitter, sweet, and astringent[20] with cooling and blunt powers and eliminates hot disorders. The roots, trunks, branches, leaves, flowers, and fruits[21] of these medicines are fragrant, attractive, and pleasing to behold, and hot disorders do not arise wherever their scent pervades.

Fragrant Mountain
To the east of that city, there is a mountain called Fragrant (Skt: *Gandhmaadan*; Tib: *sPos.Ngad lDan*), where a forest of Terminalia chebula (*A.Ru.Ra*) and Terminalia belerica (*Ba.Ru.Ra*) grows. Their roots cure bone disorders; the trunks cure muscle disorders; the branches cure disorders of blood vessels, nerves, and ligaments; the barks cure skin disorders; the leaves cure disorders of the vessel organs[22]; the flowers cure disorders of the sense organs; and the fruits cure disorders of the heart and other vital organs.[23] Five types of Terminalia chebula[24] mature atop these trees. They are endowed with the six tastes (Skt: *Rasa*; Tib: *Ro*), the eight powers (Skt: *Veerya*; Tib: *Nus.Pa*), the three post-digestive tastes (Skt: *Vipaka*; Tib: *Zhu.rJes gSum*), and the seventeen secondary qualities (Skt: *Guna*; Tib: *Yon.Tan*). These eliminate all types of disorders and are fragrant,

attractive, and pleasing to behold, and the 404 diseases will not arise wherever their scent pervades.

All of the tastes, powers, post-digestive tastes, and secondary qualities arise from 'Byung.Ba. 'Byung.Ba means to bring forth or come into existence, and this has been translated in English as "element." A verse in Tibetan by Tagtsang Lotsawa Sherab Rinchen reads:

> sNod.bCud brTan.gYo'i dNgos.Po Kun
> Sa Chu Me Rlung Nam.mKha' bCas
> 'Di.Dag La.brTen 'Byung.Ba'i Phyir
> 'Byung.Ba Zhes.Su bShad.Pa Yin

The English translation is:

> All the immobile and mobile phenomena of the world
> Are brought forth by depending on these things
> Such as Earth, Water, Fire, Air, and Space
> And thus, they are called 'Byung.Ba.

A line in Kalachakra Tantra reads:

"Ji.lTar Phyi.Rol Ji.bZhin Nang." This states that the external world reflects the internal in its composition of the five elements; as within, so without.

A verse in rGyud-bZhi reads:

> 'Gro.Ba'i Lus.'Di 'Byung.Ba bZhi.Las Grub
> gSo.Bya'i Nad.Kyang 'Byung.Ba bZhi.Yis bsKyed
> gNyen.Po'i sMan.Yang 'Byung.bZhi'i Ngo.Bo Nyid
> Lus.Nad gNyen.Po bDag.Nyid gCig.Par 'Brel

The English translation is:

> The bodies of sentient beings are composed of four elements
> The objects of healing (diseases) are caused by four elements
> And the antidotes (medicines) are also endowed with four elements
> Thus, the body, diseases, and antidotes are of same entity, i.e., the four elements.

The tastes, powers, and other qualities of the food, beverages, and medicinal substances have Earth as their basis, are moistened by Water, ripened by Fire, moved by Air, and form in Space. Though all five elements are present in them, a predominance of two of the five determines the taste. Earth and Water generate sweet; Fire and Earth sour; Water and Fire salty; Water and Air bitter; Fire and Air hot; and Earth and Air astringent.[25] Likewise, the combination of Earth and Water gives rise to *Bad.Kan*, Fire to *mKhris.Pa*, and Air to *Rlung*. The element Space is common to and pervades all other elements and *Nyes.Pa* (afflictions).

The function of the Earth element is to make the limbs firm, develop the body, and make it compact. It balances *Rlung*. Water provides moisture, softens the body, and makes it compact. It balances *mKhris.Pa*. Fire heats the body, matures the bodily constituents, and clears the complexion. It balances *Bad.Kan*. Air provides firmness and articulation of the body and distributes nutritional essences and other constituents throughout the body. It balances the combined *Bad.Kan* and *mKhris.Pa* disorders. The Space element bestows hollowness and provides extensive space. It cures the disorders of all *Nyes.Pa*.

The subtle qualities an element Earth inherits are heavy, stable, blunt, smooth, oily, and dry. Water inherits fluid, cool, heavy, blunt, oily, and flexible. Fire inherits hot, sharp, dry, coarse, light, oily, and mobile. Air inherits light, mobile, cold, coarse, non-oily, and dry. Similarly, the characteristics of *Bad.Kan* are oily, cool, heavy, blunt, smooth, stable, and sticky. The characteristics of *mKhris.Pa* are oily, sharp, hot, light, fetid, purgative, and fluid. The characteristics of *Rlung* are coarse, light, cold, subtle, hard, and mobile. The three postdigestive tastes of sweet, sour, and bitter in turn aggravate *Bad.Kan*, *mKhris.Pa*, and *Rlung* and pacify *Rlung* and *mKhris.Pa*, *Rlung* and *Bad.Kan*, and *Bad.Kan* and *mKhris.Pa* disorders. The effects of the six tastes, eight powers, and seventeen secondary qualities on the *Nyes.Pa gSum*[26] follow in the Table 1.1.4, Table 1.1.5, and Table 1.1.6.

Table 1.1.4: The Effects of the Six Tastes on the *Nyes.Pa gSum*

Tastes	Aggravates	Pacifies
Sweet (mNgar)	*Bad.Kan* disorder	*Rlung* & *mKhris.Pa* disorders
Sour (sKyur)	*mKhris.Pa* "	*Rlung* & *Bad.Kan* "
Salty (Lan.Tsha)	*mKhris.Pa* "	*Rlung* & *Bad.Kan* "
Bitter (Kha.Ba)	*Rlung* and *Bad.Kan* disorders	*mKhris.Pa* disorder
Hot (Tsha.Ba)	*mKhris.Pa* disorder	*Bad.Kan* "
Astringent (bsKa.Ba)	*Rlung* and *Bad.Kan* disorders	*mKhris.Pa* "

Table 1.1.5: The Effects of the Eight Powers on the *Nyes.Pa gSum*

Powers	Aggravates	Pacifies
Heavy (lCi.Ba)	*Bad.Kan* disorder	*Rlung* disorder
Oily (sNum.Pa)	*Bad.Kan* and *mKhris.Pa* disorders	*Rlung* "
Cool (bSil.Ba)	*Bad.Kan* and *Rlung* "	*mKhris.Pa* "
Blunt (rTul.Ba)	*Bad.Kan* disorder	*mKhris.Pa* "
Light (Yang.Ba)	*Rlung* "	*Bad.Kan* "

Coarse (rTsub.Pa)	*Rlung*	"	*Bad.Kan*	"
Hot (Tsha.Ba)	*mKhris.Pa*	"	*Bad.Kan*	"
Sharp (rNo.Ba)	*mKhris.Pa*	"	*Bad.Kan*	"

Table 1.1.6: The Effects of the seventeen Secondary Qualities on the *Nyes.Pa gSum*

Secondary Qualities	Aggravates	Pacifies
1. Smooth ('Jam.Pa)	*Bad.Kan* disorder	*Rlung* disorder
2. Heavy (lCi.Ba)	*Bad.Kan* "	" "
3. Warm (Dro.Ba)	*mKhris.Pa* "	" "
4. Oily (sNum.Pa)	*mKhris.Pa* and *Bad.Kan* disorders	" "
5. Stable (brTan.Pa)	*Bad.Kan* disorders	" "
6. Cold (Grang.Ba)	*Rlung* and *Bad.Kan* disorders	*mKhris.Pa* disorder
7. Blunt (rTul.Ba)	*Bad.Kan* disorder	" "
8. Cool (bSil.Ba)	*Rlung* and *Bad.Kan* disorders	" "
9. Flexible (mNyen.Pa)	*Bad.Kan* disorder	" "
10. Fluid (sLa.Ba)	*Bad.Kan* "	" "
11. Dry (sKam.Pa)	*Rlung* "	" "
12. Non-oily (sKya.Ba)	*Rlung* "	*Bad.Kan* disorder
13. Hot (Tsha.Ba)	*mKhris.Pa* "	" "
14. Light (Yang.Ba)	*Rlung* and *mKhris.Pa* disorders	" "
15. Sharp (rNo.Ba)	*mKhris.Pa* disorder	" "
16. Coarse (rTsub.Ba)	*Rlung* "	" "
17. Mobile (gYo.Ba)	*Rlung* "	" "

Garlanded Mountain

To the west of that city, there is a mountain called Garlanded (Skt: *Malaya*; Tib: *Phreng.lDan*), where six good medicines grow. These are nutmeg (*Dza'.Ti*), Bambusa textilis (*Cu.Gang*), saffron (*Gur.Gum*), Amomum subulatum (*Ka.Ko.La*), cardamom (*Sug.sMel*), and clove (*Li.Shi*). With respect to the organs, they are good for the disorders of heart, lungs, liver, spleen, kidneys, and life vessels, [27] respectively. They are also considered good for the disorders of *Rlung*, *mKhris.Pa*, *mKhris.Pa*, *Bad.Kan*, *Bad.Kan*, and *Rlung*, respectively. This mountain is endowed with the five kinds of calcite (*Cong.Zhi*), [28] the five kinds of mineral exudate (*Brag.Zhun*), [29] the five kinds of medicinal waters, and the five kinds of hot springs which pacify all disorders. See the Table 1.1.7 below for the qualities of the five kinds of medicinal waters.

Table 1.1.7: The Five Kinds of Medicinal Waters

Taste	Color of Algae	Power	Pacifies
1. Sweet	Bluish	Heavy and smooth	*Rlung* disorder

2. Bitter	Yellowish	Blunt	*mKhris.Pa* disorder and (laxative)
3. Sour	Whitish	Coarse and sharp	*Bad.Kan* disorder and (expectorant)
4. Sweet to bitter to sour	Like a peacock's feather	Heavy, blunt, and Sharp	*Tri-Nyes.Pa* disorders
5. Sweet to bitter	Mixture of blue and yellow	Smooth and fluid	*Rlung* & *mKhris.Pa* disorders
6. Bitter to sour	Mixture of red and yellow	Blunt and sharp	*mKhris.Pa* & *Bad.Kan* disorders
7. Sweet to sour	Mixture of blue and white	Heavy, sharp, and smooth	*Bad.Kan* & *Rlung* disorders

Note that since (5) the *Rlung* and *mKhris.Pa*, (6) *Bad.Kan* and *mKhris.Pa*, and (7) *Bad.Kan* and *Rlung* combined disorders are of dual combinations, they are counted as one.

Another version of the five medicinal waters' effects is based solely on their tastes and their origination from areas where calcite is found. The medicinal waters tasting sour and salty, sour and sweet, sour and hot, sour and bitter, and sour and astringent pacify *Bad.Kan* and *Rlung*, *Bad.Kan* and *mKhris.Pa*, *Bad.Kan*, *Bad.Kan* and blood, and *Bad.Kan sMug.Po*[30] disorders, respectively.

The five kinds of hot springs are:

(1) The hot springs in areas of coal (*rDo.Sol*) and calcite eliminate hot disorders.

(2) The hot springs in areas of coal and sulphur (*Mu.Zi*) alleviate lymph and cold disorders but aggravate *Rlung* because of their coarse power.

(3) The hot spring coming from the area of coal and mineral exudate is neutral in power and eliminates the combination of dual and *tri-Nyes.Pa* disorders.

(4) The hot spring coming from the area of coal, calcite, and sulphur eliminates cold disorders.

(5) The hot spring coming from the area of coal, sulphur, mineral exudates, and realgar (*lDong.Ros*) eliminates lymph and hot disorders.

The surroundings of the city are meadow of saffron with the wafting of its fragrance, and all the rocks are endowed with all kinds of mineral medicines and salts. Atop the trees in the forest of medicine, peacock, *Shang.Shang*,[31] and parrot birds sing sweetly, and on the ground aside are elephant, bear, and musk deer, animals bearing good medicines on their body.

In summary, in *lTa.Na.sDug*, grows all kinds of medicines and hence there is nothing the medicinal substances have not adorned it.

Excellent Teacher

In the center of that palace, Master, the Victorious Conqueror, Healer, Supreme Physician, King of Vaidurya Light sat on a jewel throne made of yellow, white, and blue Vaidurya. The appearance of Medicine Buddha[32]could be understood from the following Tibetan verse.

> *Rigs.Kyi gTso.Bo bCom.lDan sMan.rGyal mThing*
> *mTshan.dPe'i rGyan.rDzogs sMan.mChog Lhung.bZed bsNams*
> *Don.gNyis mThar.Phyin Ye.Shes lNga.rDzogs dPal*
> *Dug.lNga rGyu.'Bras Nad.Sel dBang.bsKur Ro.*

The English translation is:

> The Victorious Conqueror, King of Physician, Chief of Family is blue
> Perfectly endowed with major and minor marks,[33] hold a supreme medicine,[34] and begging bowl
> Having achieved the two ultimate goals,[35] glorious and perfectly endowed with five wisdoms[36]
> Will bestow empowerment in eliminating the diseases of five poisons (cause) and its effect.[37]

The Master's radiant body is azure blue with the thirty-two marks of perfection and the eighty signs of great beauty which characterize all Buddhas. His left hand is in the gesture of meditation mudra and he holds a begging bowl full of long-life nectar, which symbolizes immortality. In his right hand he holds the "supreme medicine" (Terminalia chebula) outstretched in the gesture of supreme generosity mudra. This symbolizes giving protection from illness as well as physical and mental well-being. His abode is in the eastern direction and is called a "Light of Vaidurya." See Figure 1.1.1 below for Medicine Buddha.

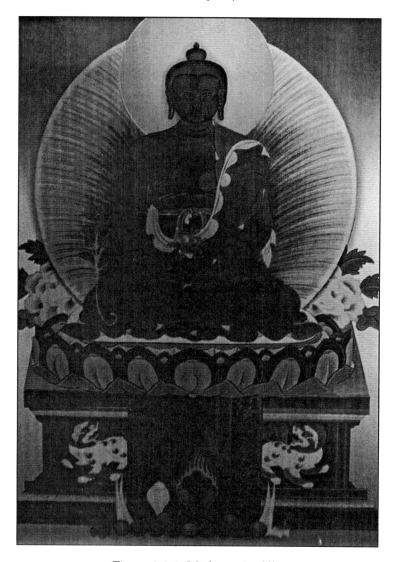

Figure 1.1.1: Medicine Buddha

Excellent Retinue

The Master is completely surrounded by four groups of disciples, gods, sages, non-Buddhists, and Buddhists. The group of gods include the celestial physician Daksha Prajapati (*sKye.rGu'i bDag.Po Myur.Ba*) [38] and Ashwini Kumaradvya (Tib: *Tha.sKar Gyi Bu.gNyis*; Eng: the two sons of Ashwini), the divine lord Indra (*Lha.'i dBang.Po brGya.Byin*), and the goddess Amrtavati (*bDud.rTsi.Ma*), [39] and many other divine disciples have gathered there.

The group of sages include the great sage the son of Atreya (*rGyun.Shes Kyi Bu*), Agnivesa (*Me.bZhin 'Jug*), Nimindhara (*Mu.Khyud 'Dzin*), son of '*Gro.Ba sKyong*, Haladhara (*gShol.'Gro sKyes*), *dKa'.gNyis sPyod*, Dhanvantari (*Thang.La.'Bar*), and Punarvasu (*Nabs.So sKyes*), and many other sages have gathered there.

The group of non-Buddhists include Brahma, the patriarch of the tirthikas (*Mu.sTegs Kyi Mes.Po Tshangs.Pa*), Mahadeva Shri Jatanika 'Shiva' (Tib: *Lha Chen.Po dPal.Gyi Ral.Pa Can*; Eng: the glorious and great god with matted hair), Vishnu (Tib: *Khyab.'Jug*; Eng: the all pervading one), and Kumara Shadanan (Tib: *gZhon.Nu gDong.Drug*; Eng: son with six faces),[40] and many other tirthikas have gathered there.

The group of Buddhists include Arya Manjushri (*'Phags.Pa 'Jam.dPal*), an embodiment of all the Buddha's wisdom aspect; Avalokiteshvara (*sPyan.Ras.gZigs dBang.Phyug*), an embodiment of all the Buddha's compassion aspect; Vajra Pani (*Phyag.Na rDo.rJe*), an embodiment of all the Buddha's might and power aspect;[41] Ananda (*Kun.dGa'.Bo*);[42] and Kumara Jivaka (*'Tso.Byed gZhon.Nu*),[43] and many other Buddhists have gathered there.

Excellent Period

The phrase "at that time" is referred to as denoting an excellent period. However, all the major commentaries on *rGyud.bZhi* quote this as a period when the Victorious Conqueror, Master of Medicine, King of Vaidurya Light, and sage *Yid.Las sKyes*, and four groups of disciples have assembled together at the City of Medicine, called *lTa.Na.sDug*.

The Elder Yuthog Yonten Gonpo (AD 708-833) had specified this in his biography as Wood male Rat years (*Shing.Pho Byi.Ba Lo*), second Tibetan month (*Cho.'Phrul Khra.Yi Zla.Ba*; Western month: March), and on the first day (*Tses.Zhag gCig.Gi Nyin.Par*)[44] Buddha Shakya Muni manifested himself in the form of Medicine Buddha and expounded the *rGyud.bZhi*.

Excellent Teaching

At that time the teachings Master gave were understood by each of the four group of disciples as tradition of one's own master.[45] Thus, this specified teaching is called a tradition of sage[46] as one's body, speech, and mind have been straightened and freed from faults as well as pacified with the imbalances of *Nyes.Pa* of others. This concludes the first chapter, the basis of discussion from the Secret Oral Instructions Tantra on the Eight Branches of the Essence of Nectar.

CHAPTER TWO

ENUMERATION OF THE SUBJECT OF DISCUSSION

At that time the master, Victorious Conqueror, Healer, Supreme Physician, the King of Vaidurya Light sat in a meditation called "King of Medicine[1]" which pacifies the 404 diseases. Immediately after entering in this absorption, from his heart several hundred thousand variegated light rays were emitted to the ten directions[2]. This removed the mental defilements[3] of sentient beings[4] in the ten directions and particularly pacified the three poisons arising from ignorance as well as their respective disorders of *Nyes.Pa gSum*. After withdrawing these (light rays) back to the heart, from his heart emanated a Master named sage *Rig.Pa'i Ye.Shes* (Skt: *Vidyajnana;* Eng: Wisdom of Awareness). The appearance of sage *Rig.Pa'i Ye.Shes* could be understood from the following Tibetan verse.

Thugs.sPrul Mi.bsKyod Rig.Pa'i Ye.Shes mThing
mTshan.dPe'i rGyan.rDzogs rDo.rJe Lhung.bZed bsNams
rTsa.rGyud sTon.mDzad Me.Long Ye.Shes Dang
Zhe.sDang rGyu.'Bras Nad.Sel dBang.bsKur Ro.

The English translation is:

The heart emanation Aprakampa,[5] *Rig.Pa'i Ye.Shes* is blue
Perfectly adorned with major and minor marks, hold a vajra and begging bowl
Expounding the Root Tantra, will bestow the empowerment
Of mirror-like wisdom and in eliminating the cause and effect of anger.

The sage's radiant body is azure blue, and in his left hand, he holds a begging bowl full of long-life nectar. In his right hand, he holds a vajra. He appeared in space in front of Medicine Buddha and welcomed the sages and disciples by saying, "Oh friends, (you) must know this. One who desires to be remaining free from sickness as well as wants to heal the sickness should learn the oral instructions of the Science of Healing. One who desires a long life should learn the oral instructions of the Science of Healing. One who desires to receive teachings, wealth, and happiness should learn the oral instructions of the Science of Healing. One who desires to liberate[6] self and others from the anguish of three mental poisons and the disorders of *Nyes.Pa gSum* and wants regard and respect from others should learn the oral instructions of the Science of Healing."

Thus he had spoken these words, from the tongue of the Master, King of Vaidurya Light, several hundred thousand variegated light rays were emitted to the ten directions. These (light rays) removed the verbal defilements[7] of sentient beings in the ten directions and particularly pacified the disorders of *Nyes.Pa gSum* and harmful influences from evil spirits. After withdrawing these (light rays) back to the tongue, sage *Yid.Las sKyes* (Skt: *Manasija*; Eng: Born from the Mind), an emanation of speech appeared. The appearance of sage *Yid.Las sKyes* could be understood from following Tibetan verse.

gSung.sPrul mTha'Yas Yid.Las sKyes.Pa dMar
mTshan.dPe'i rGyan.rDzogs Pad.Ma Lhung.bZed bsNams
rGyud.Kyi Zhu.Chen Sor.rTog Ye.Shes Dang
'Dod.Chags rGyu.'Bras Nad.Sel dBang.bsKur Ro.

The English translation is:

The speech emanation Amitabha,[8] *Yid.Las sKyes* is red
Perfectly adorned with major and minor marks, hold a padma and begging bowl
Great petitioner of tantra, would bestow the empowerment
Of discriminating wisdom and in eliminating the cause and effect of attachment.

The sage's radiant body is red, and in his left hand, he holds a begging bowl full of long-life nectar. In his right hand, he holds a lotus flower. After doing prostration and circumambulation to the Master, sage *Yid.Las sKyes* sat in front of the Master in a manner of lion watching.[9] He then made a request to the Master on behalf of sages and other disciples, "Oh Master, sage *Rig.Pa'i Ye.Shes*, as we aspire to fulfill the sublime purpose of self and others, how may we learn the oral instructions of the Science of Healing?"

Thus, after the request, the mind emanation, sage *Rig.Pa'i Ye.Shes* replied, "Oh great sage, learn the oral instructions tantra of the Science of Healing. Learn the branches. Learn the principles. Learn the divisions. Learn the compilations. Learn the chapters."

After he had spoken that, the sage *Yid.Las sKyes* requested, "How may we learn the oral instruction's tantra of the Science of Healing?" The Master replied, "Oh great sage, listen. Learn the *rGyud.bZhi* (Four Tantras). The sage *Rig.Pa'i Ye.Shes* then unfolds the classifications of the Four Tantras, the eight branches, the eleven principles, the fifteen divisions, the four compilations, and the chapters of the Four Tantras in successive order."

See the Table 1.2.1 below for Four Tantras.

Table 1.2.1: The Four Tantras

Tantra	No. of Chapters	No. of Verses
rTsa.rGyud (Root Tantra)	6	120
bShad.rGyud (Explanatory Tantra)	31	773 1/2
Man.Ngag rGyud (Oral Instructions Tantra)	92	4028
Phyi.Ma rGyud (Last Tantra)	27	1014
Total	156	5935 1/2

It is said that the reasons behind expounding the Root, Explanatory, Oral Instructions, and Last Tantra are based on the level of a person's intelligence, i.e., sharp, moderate, poor, and very poor, respectively.

The Eight Branches

See the explanation about the eight branches in Part One, Chapter One, Basis of Discussion under *Yan.Lag brGyad.Pa* (the explanation of the title in Tibetan follows in order) and the Notes number four of the same chapter and at the end of this chapter.

The Eleven Principles

Learn the eleven principles (*gNas bCu.gCig*):

(1) The principle of the concise of fundamentals
(2) The principle of the formation of body
(3) The principle of the waxing and waning of *Nyes.Pa*
(4) The principle of the pattern of behavior
(5) The principle of the dietetics
(6) The principle of the compounding of medicines
(7) The principle of the therapeutic instruments
(8) The principle of the disease-free normal health
(9) The principle of the techniques of diagnosis
(10) The principle of the healing techniques
(11) The principle of the code and conduct of physician

The Fifteen Divisions

Learn the fifteen divisions (*sKabs bCo.lNga*):

(1) The division of healing *Nyes.Pa* gSum
(2) The division of healing internal disorders
(3) The division of healing fevers
(4) The division of healing upper body disorders
(5) The division of healing the diseases of vital and vessel organs
(6) The division of healing secret (genital) disorders
(7) The division of healing miscellaneous disorders
(8) The division of healing secondary sores
(9) The division of healing children's diseases
(10) The division of healing female's diseases
(11) The division of healing diseases caused by evil spirits
(12) The division of healing wounds inflicted by weapons
(13) The division of healing the diseases caused by poisons
(14) The division of healing old age diseases
(15) The division of healing impotency

The Four Compilations

Learn the four compilations (*mDo.bZhi*):

(1) The compilation of pulse and urine examination
(2) The compilation of pacification medicines[10]
(3) The compilation of cleansing works[11]
(4) The compilation of smooth and coarse accessory therapy.[12]

The Six Chapters of Root Tantra

Learn the 156 chapters beginning with the chapters of Root Tantra:

(1) The basis of discussion
(2) The enumeration of the subject of discussion
(3) The basis of normal and abnormal body
(4) Diagnosis
(5) Methods of healing
(6) Summary of Root Tantra is to be understood in the synthesis of principle of Root Tantra

The Thirty-One Chapters of Explanatory Tantra

The chapters of Explanatory Tantra are:

(1) Summary of Explanatory Tantra
(2) Embryology

(3) The similes of the body
(4) Anatomy
(5) Physiology
(6) Function and classification of the body
(7) Signs of death
(8) Primordial causes of disorders
(9) Immediate causes of disorders
(10) The modes of entering diseases
(11) The characteristics of *Rlung, mKhris.Pa*, and *Bad.Kan* disorders
(12) Classification of disease
(13) The routine behavior
(14) Seasonal behavior
(15) Incidental behavior
(16) Dietetics
(17) Dietary restrictions
(18) Dietary regimen dealing with moderate intake of food and drinks
(19) The taste and post-digestive (taste)
(20) The inherent powers of medicinal substances
(21) The categories and methods of compounding medicines
(22) Therapeutic instruments
(23) Remaining abiding healthy
(24) General techniques for correct diagnosis
(25) Techniques for gaining patients' confidence
(26) Four diagnostic techniques[13] to verify whether or not the patient is curable
(27) General healing techniques
(28) Specific healing techniques
(29) Two healing techniques
(30) The actual healing techniques for *Nyes.Pa*
(31) The code and conduct of the physician

Three single chapters are therapeutic instruments (22); remaining abiding healthy (23); and the code and conduct of the physician (31). Four sets of three chapters are pattern of behavior (13, 14, 15); dietetics (16, 17, 18); compounding medicines (19, 20, 21); and techniques of diagnosis (22, 23, 24). One set of four chapters is healing techniques (27, 28, 29, 30); one set of five chapters is waxing and waning of *Nyes.Pa* (8, 9, 10, 11, 12); and one set of six chapters is the formation of body (2, 3, 4, 5, 6, 7). Plus the summary of Explanatory Tantra (1), make thirty-one chapters in all.

The Ninety-Two Chapters of Oral Instruction's Tantra

The chapters of Oral Instruction's Tantra are:
(1) Requesting to expound the Oral Instruction's Tantra

(2) Healing of *Rlung* disorders

(3) Healing of *mKhris.Pa* disorders

(4) Healing of *Bad.Kan* disorders

(5) Healing of *Bad.Kan sMug.Po*

(6) Healing of indigestion, the cause of all internal disorders

(7) Healing of internal tumors

(8) Healing of initial stage edema

(9) Healing of second stage edema[14]

(10) Healing of last stage edema[15]

(11) Healing of chronic wasting disease

(12) Healing of general fever

(13) Clearing the basis of errors on contra indications of hot and cold disorders

(14) The junction of fever between mountain and plain[16]

(15) Healing of unripened fever[17]

(16) Healing of high fever

(17) Healing of empty fever[18]

(18) Healing of hidden fever[19]

(19) Healing of chronic fever

(20) Healing of complicated fever[20]

(21) Healing of spread fever[21]

(22) Healing of disturbed fever[22]

(23) Healing of epidemic fever

(24) Healing of small pox

(25) Healing of dysentery

(26) Healing of inflammation associated with throat and muscles

(27) Healing of common cold

(28) Healing of diseases of the head

(29) Healing of diseases of the eyes

(30) Healing of diseases of the ears

(31) Healing of diseases of the nose

(32) Healing of diseases of the mouth

(33) Healing of goiters

(34) Healing of heart diseases

(35) Healing of lung diseases

(36) Healing of liver diseases

(37) Healing of spleen diseases

(38) Healing of renal diseases

(39) Healing of diseases of the stomach

(40) Healing of diseases of the small intestine

(41) Healing of diseases of the large intestine

(42) Healing of diseases of the male organ

(43) Healing of diseases of the female organ

(44) Healing of vocal obstruction

(45) Healing of anorexia

(46) Healing of excessive thirst

(47) Healing of hiccup

(48) Healing of asthma

(49) Healing of sudden abdominal cramps

(50) Healing of disorders caused by micro-organisms

(51) Healing of vomiting

(52) Healing of diarrhea

(53) Healing of constipation

(54) Healing of obstruction of the urine

(55) Healing of frequent urination[23]

(56) Healing of diarrhea caused by intestinal fever

(57) Healing of gout

(58) Healing of arthritis

(59) Healing of lymph disorders

(60) Healing of neurological disorders

(61) Healing of skin diseases

(62) Healing of miscellaneous minor disorders[24]

(63) Healing of malignant tumors[25]

(64) Healing of hemorrhoids

(65) Healing of erysipelas

(66) Healing of abscess[26]

(67) Healing of lymphadenopathy

(68) Healing of swelling of the testicles[27]

(69) Healing of rKang.'Bam[28]

(70) Healing of anal fistula

(71) Care of children in proper environment

(72) Healing of diseases of the children

(73) Healing of childrens' diseases caused by evil spirits

(74) Healing of chief general gynecological diseases[29]

(75) Healing of specific gynecological diseases[30]

(76) Healing of common gynecological diseases[31]

(77) Healing of diseases caused by elemental spirits[32]

(78) Healing of insanity[33]

(79) Healing of amnesia[34]

(80) Healing of planetary-spirit-caused disorders[35]

(81) Healing of mischievous serpent-spirit-caused diseases[36]

(82) Healing of general wounds

(83) Healing of head wounds

(84) Healing of neck wounds

(85) Healing of upper and lower abdominal wounds

(86) Healing of limb wounds

(87) Healing of diseases caused by compounded poisons

(88) Healing of food poisoning
(89) Healing of diseases caused by movable and immovable poisons[37]
(90) Healing of old age disorders by rejuvenation
(91) Healing the sexual drive and sperm
(92) Healing of infertility in women

Thus, the single chapter is old age disorders (90); and two sets of two chapters are secret (genital) disorders (42, 43) and impotency (91, 92). Three sets of three chapters are childrens' diseases (71, 72, 73); gynecological diseases (74, 75, 76); and diseases related to toxics (87, 88, 89). One set of four chapters is disorders of Nyes.Pa gSum (2, 3, 4, 5); and two sets of five chapters are evil-spirit-caused diseases (77, 78, 79, 80, 81) and wounds inflicted by weapons (82, 83, 84, 85, 86). Two sets of six chapters are internal disorders (6, 7, 8, 9, 10, 11) and upper body disorders (28, 29, 30, 31, 32, 33). Two sets of eight chapters are diseases of the vital and vessel organs (34, 35, 36, 37, 38, 39, 40, 41) and secondary sores (63, 64, 65, 66, 67, 68, 69, 70). One set of sixteen chapters is fever (12 to 27) and one set of nineteen chapters are miscellaneous disorders (44 to 62). Plus requesting to expound the Oral Instruction's Tantra (1), make ninety-two chapters in all.

The Twenty-Five Chapters of Last Tantra

The chapters of Last Tantra are:

(1) The pulse examination
(2) The urine examination
(3) Category of decoctions[38]
(4) Category of powders[39]
(5) Category of pills[40]
(6) Category of paste[41]
(7) Category of medicinal butters[42]
(8) Category of calcinated medicines[43]
(9) Category of concentrated decoctions[44]
(10) Category of medicinal chang (wine)[45]
(11) Category of jewel compounds[46]
(12) Category of herbal compounds[47]
(13) Preliminary oil therapy for five cleansing works[48]
(14) Purgatives
(15) Emetics
(16) Nasal medications[49]
(17) Mild suppositories
(18) Enema[50]
(19) Vessel cleansing therapy[51]
(20) Venesection

(21) Moxibustions
(22) Compress therapy
(23) Medicinal bath therapy[52]
(24) Massage therapy[53]
(25) Spoon surgical techniques.[54]

One set of two chapters is pulse examination (1) and urine examination (2); one set of ten chapters is pacification medicines (3 to 12); one set of seven chapters is cleansing works (13 to 19); and one set of six chapters is smooth and coarse accessory therapy (20 to 25).

Thus, there are 154 chapters in *rGyud.bZhi*, plus the concluding and the entrustment of entire tantras; the overall total is 156 chapters. The eight branches are explained disorderly in the first, second, and fourth tantras, whereas the third tantra (Oral Instruction's Tantra) provides them in a systematic order. Thus, there are seventy chapters on *Lus*; three chapters each on *Byis.Pa*, *Mo.Nad*, and *Dug*; five chapters each on *gDon* and *mTshon*; one chapter on *rGas*; and two chapters on *Ro.Tsa*. In total there are ninety-two chapters. This concludes the second chapter, the enumeration of the subject of discussion from the Secret Oral Instruction's Tantra on the Eight Branches of the Essence of Nectar.

CHAPTER THREE

THE BASIS OF NORMAL AND ABNORMAL BODY

Immediately following the teachings of Chapter Two, the sage *Yid.Las sKyes* requested to the sage *Rig.Pa'i Ye.Shes*, "Oh Master, sage *Rig.Pa'i Ye.Shes Lags[1]*, from the four types of tantra on the Science of Healing how may (we[2]) learn the Root Tantra? Healer, King of physicians, please expound." Then the mind emanation, sage *Rig.Pa'i Ye.Shes* replied to his disciple, "Oh Great sage *Yid.Las sKyes*, (I shall) first explain the concise principles of Root Tantra. On 3 roots, grow 9 trunks, out of which spread 47 branches, which develop 224 leaves. Atop the first trunk sit two blossoms and three ripened fruits.[3]" (The explanation also appears in the summary of the Root Tantra. Refer to Part One, Chapter 6.)

The Great Master then began with the topic of the basis of the normal and abnormal body referring to the Allegorical Tree (see Figure 1.3.1) as it represents the human body. The body has three aspects: the *Nyes.Pa* (humors[4]), the bodily constituents, and the excretions. Their normal and abnormal states maintain health and afflict the body, respectively.

Table 1.3.1 summarizes the number of trunks, branches, leaves, flowers, and fruits discussed in this chapter.

Table 1.3.1: The Root of the Normal and Abnormal Body

Trunk No.	Branches	Leaves	Flowers	Fruits
Normal	3	25	2	3
Abnormal	9	63	-	-
Total	12	88	2	3

Two trunks grow from the root of the body. The first trunk deals with the normal mind-body in a state of dynamic equilibrium, while the second trunk deals with the abnormal mind-body in an abnormal state.

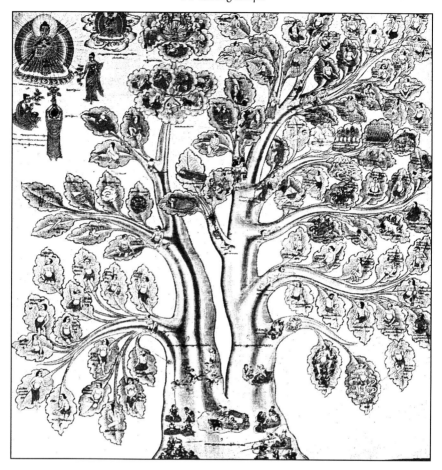

Figure 1.3.1: Allegorical Tree of the Normal and Abnormal Body

Trunk Number One

Trunk Number One represents the normal body and on it spreads the branches of *Nyes.Pa*, bodily constituents and excretions. On these branches, in turn, grow fifteen, seven, and three leaves. As mentioned earlier, the dynamic equilibrium of these twenty-five leaves ensure normal function of the mind-body as well as general well being. The disruption of this equilibrium results in ill health. A sequential explanation of each of these leaves follows.

Note: Tibetan medicine is traditionally memorized by its practitioners using numerical cues for the different concepts. These numbers are listed consecutively in parentheses and italics throughout this chapter.

Branch 1: Fifteen Afflictions (Nyes.Pa bCo.lNga)

The Five Subdivisions of *Rlung*

The next five items are the subdivisions of *Rlung*, along with their locations and functions. In general, *Rlung* is responsible for exhalation and inhalation and for physical, verbal, and mental activities. It travels through the objects of harm and enables urination, defecation, menstruation, development and delivery of the fetus, spitting, belching, and speech. *Rlung* also ensures the clarity of the mental and sense organs and sustains the body.

(1) **Rlung Srog.'Dzin** (Life sustaining *Rlung*)
Location:	Crown of head[5]
Passage:	Pharynx and esophagus
Action:	Swallowing of food and drink, inhaling, spitting, sneezing and belching, clears the perceptions of sense organs and the mind as well as integrating the mind and body.

(2) **Rlung Gyen.rGyu** (Ascending *Rlung*)
Location:	Chest[6]
Passage:	Nostrils, tongue, and throat
Action:	Speech, clear complexion, regulation of body color, physical strength, clarity of memory, and diligence.

(3) **Rlung Khyab.Byed** (Pervasive *Rlung*)
Location:	Heart
Passage:	Circulates in all the blood vessels of body
Action:	Proper function of muscles, lifting, walking, stretching, contraction, opening and closing of orifices; most of the physical, verbal, and mental functions depend on this.

(4) **Rlung Me.mNyam** (Fire accompanying *Rlung*)
Location:	*Pho.Ba*[7]
Passage:	Throughout the alimentary canal
Action:	Assists in digestion, separates the nutrients and waste products, and ripens the successive objects of harm.[8]

(5) **Rlung Thur.Sel** (Downward voiding *Rlung*)
Location:	Anal canal[9]
Passage:	Large intestine, urinary *bladder*, reproductive organs and thighs

Action: Assists in holding and releasing of feces, urine, sperm, menstrual blood, and ovum; retaining and delivering a child and the placenta.

The Five Subdivisions of *mKhris.Pa*

The next five items are the subdivisions of *mKhris.Pa*, along with their locations and functions. In general, *mKhris.Pa* causes hunger, thirst, appetite, and digestion, and promotes bodily heat, complexion, courage, and intelligence.

(6) **mKhris.Pa 'Ju.Byed** (Digestive *mKhris.Pa*)
Location: Between the digested and undigested part of *Pho.Ba*[10]
Action: Responsible for main digestion, separation of some nutrients and waste products, greatly promotes the warmth of the body, assists and empowers the functioning of the remaining four types of *mKhris.Pa*.

(7) **mKhris.Pa mDangs.sGyur** (Complexion transforming *mKhris.Pa*)[11]
Location: Liver
Action: Responsible for transformation of blood and muscles to redness.

(8) **mKhris.Pa sGrub.Byed** (Accomplishing *mKhris.Pa*)
Location: Heart
Action: Responsible for clear and quick recollection, pride, and diligence in accomplishing one's desire.

(9) **mKhris.Pa mThong.Byed** (Sight *mKhris.Pa*)
Location: Eyes
Action: Responsible for seeing diverse objects.

(10) **mKhris.Pa mDog.gSal** (Color clearing *mKhris.Pa*)
Location: Skin
Action: Responsible for clear and bright skin color.

The Five Subdivisions of *Bad.Kan*

The next five items are the subdivisions of *Bad.Kan* along with their locations and functions. In general, *Bad.Kan* is responsible for firmness and stability of both body and mind, inducing sleep, connecting the body joints, inducing tolerance, lubricating the internal systems, and ensuring skin smoothness.

(11) Bad.Kan rTen.Byed (Supporting *Bad.Kan*)

Location:	Chest[12]
Action:	Supports the remaining four types of *Bad.Kan*, quenches thirst though one has not drunk liquid, and functions similarly to that of the body's fluid system.

(12) Bad.Kan Myag.Byed (Decomposing *Bad.Kan*)

Location:	Undigested part of *Pho.Ba*[13]
Action:	Responsible for decomposing and blending of ingested foodstuffs with fluid to form a semi-liquid.

(13) Bad.Kan Myong.Byed (Experiencing *Bad.Kan*)

Location:	Tongue
Action:	Responsible for capturing six tastes.

(14) Bad.Kan Tshim.Byed (Satisfying *Bad.Kan*) [14]

Location:	Head[15]
Action:	Responsible for satisfaction as well as empowering the function of the five sense organ's functions.

(15) Bad.Kan 'Byor.Byed (Connecting *Bad.Kan*)

Location:	In all the joints of body
Action:	Connects joints and assists in stretching and contracting the limbs.

Branch 2: Seven Bodily Constituents (Lus.Zungs bDun)

Now in Branch 2, the next seven bodily constituents are like the building materials that support life. The proper functions of *Nyes.Pa*, particularly the digestive heats, create the seven bodily constituents, which are called *Lus.Zungs bDun* in Tibetan. The sources of the seven bodily constituents are ingested foods and beverages. Each successive sequence of the post-nutritional essences takes one day to form its essence. Hence, to produce a regenerative fluid, it takes six days.

(16) Dangs.Ma (Nutritional essence):

Formed from:	ingested foodstuffs

(17) Khrag (Blood):

Formed from:	the essence of *Dangs.Ma*

(18) Sha (Muscles):

Formed from:	the essence of blood

(19) Tshil (Fats):

Formed from:	the essence of muscles

(20) Rus (Bones):

Formed from: the essence of fats

(21) *rKang* (Marrow):

Formed from: the essence of bones

(22) **Khu.Ba** (Regenerative fluid):

Formed from: the essence of marrow

Branch 3: Three Excretions (Dri.Ma gSum)

(23) **bShang.Ba** (Feces):

Function: To support the ingested foodstuffs, decompose and transform them into feces, and then evacuate from the anal region.

(24) **gCin** (Urine):

Function: To support the body's fluids, transform them into urine, and then evacuate them from the bladder.

(25) **rNgul** (Perspiration):

Function: To soften the skin, unblock the pores, and to stabilize body hair.

Two Flowers

(1) **Nad Med.pa** (Freedom from disease)
(2) **Tshe Ring.Ba** (Long life)

Three Fruits

As a result of the above two blossoms, the following mature:

(1) **Chos** (High spiritual life):

Symbolizes: Temporal knowledge of worldly and religious activities, rich in the seven noble wealths[16] (qualities) and happiness in this life

(2) **Nor** (Wealth):

Symbolizes: Abundance of material possessions (jewels and garments, etc.)

(3) **bDe.Ba** (Happiness):

Symbolizes: Ultimate happiness, represented by the liberation of body in a cross-legged sitting posture and transference of consciousness to a paradise with hoisting of an umbrella by gods and goddesses.

Trunk Number Two

Trunk Number Two represents the abnormal body in nine branches: the primary causes of *Nyes.Pa*, the immediate causes, general passages, general locations, the progression of *Nyes.Pa*, period of manifestation of *Nyes.Pa*, disorders of terminal effects, causes of adverse reactions, and summation. On these branches, in turn, grow three, four, six, three, fifteen, nine, nine, twelve, and two leaves and their explanation follows in successive order. Table 1.3.2 identifies the *Nyes.Pa* that arises from mental poisons.

Table 1.3.2: The Mental Poisons and *Nyes.Pa* gSum

Root Cause (Mental)	Specific Cause (Mental)	Location	Nyes.Pa Cause (Closest Physical)
Ma.Rig.Pa (Ignorance)	gTi.Mug	Brain	*Bad.Kan*
	Zhe.sDang	Liver/Gall *bladder*	*mKhris.Pa*
	'Dod.Chags	Genital organs	*Rlung*

Branch 1: The Primary Causes of Nyes.Pa

(1) **'Dod.Chags** (Attachment): gives rise to *Rlung*
(2) **Zhe.sDang** (Anger): gives rise to *mKhris.Pa*
(3) **gTi.Mug** (Delusion): gives rise to *Bad.Kan*

In the tree illustration, these aspects are represented by a couple having sex, two people quarrelling, and a person in deep sleep, respectively. In the "Wheel of Life," a peacock, a snake, and a pig denote these (respectively).

The root cause of all suffering and misapprehension (wrong view) has been traced to *Ma.Rig.Pa* (Ignorance/Unawareness).[17] It prevents the mind from understanding the law of causality and recognizing the reality of phenomena. This, in turn, gives rise to *'Dod.Chags*, *Zhe.sDang*, and *gTi.Mug*, whose respective effects are *Rlung*, *mKhris.Pa*, and *Bad.Kan*.

When intense, *gTi.Mug*, a negative mental factor that is heavy, dull, and cloudy, can increase *Bad.Kan*. *Bad.Kan*, possessing similar characteristics when manifested in the brain, can decrease intelligence and obscure clarity, leading to confusion.

Zhe.sDang, when intense, causes disturbances from the middle part of the body. Blood, being warm, relates to both *Zhe.sDang* and *mKhris.Pa*, and flows in the *Srog.rTsa Nag.Po* (black life vessel).[18] *mKhris.Pa*, which is hot and burns like a fire when increased in the liver and gall *bladder*, induces body heat to the point where it destroys the bodily constituents.

'Dod.Chags, which is light and mobile, corresponds to the characteristics of *Rlung*. Since regenerative fluids relate to both *'Dod.Chags* and *Rlung*, *'Dod.Chags*

therefore abides in the genital organs. When intense, it increases attraction toward the opposite sex. This attraction generates more and more eagerness, gradually leading to emotional anxiety, paving the way for the rise of *Rlung* disorders. *Rlung* imbalances emanate from the lower part of the body, particularly the hips and waist.

Branch 2: The Immediate Causes of Nyes.Pa

(4) Seasonal changes: Inadequate, excessive, or inappropriate behavior with relation to the season
Example: A person living naked during the winter[19]
(5) Evil spirits:
Example: The devil or a malicious king spirit, inflicting harm
(6) Unwholesome diet:
Example: Improper intake of meat and alcohol (both produce heat) in the sun
(7) Inappropriate behavior:
Example: Abiding in the sun wearing fur clothes during *Sos.Ka* (early summer)

Branch 3: General Passages of Nyes.Pa[20]

The imbalances raised by the previous four factors (4-7) cause *Nyes.Pa* to operate in a sequence.

Nyes.Pa:
(8) Spreads on the skin
(9) Develops in the muscles
(10) Moves through the vessels (blood vessels and nerves)
(11) Affects the bones
(12) Descends to *Don.lNga* (five vital organs)
(13) Falls into the *sNod.Drug* (six vessel organs)

Branch 4: General Locations of Nyes.Pa

(14) *Bad.Kan* is located in the upper part of the body.
(15) *mKhris.Pa* is located in the middle part of the body.
(16) *Rlung* is located in the lower part of the body.
For details, see Table 1.3.2.

Branch 5: The Progression of Nyes.Pa[21]

Rlung then progresses in the:

(17) Bones (bodily constituents)
(18) Ears (sense organs)
(19) Pores and skin surface (belongs to excretion)
(20) Heart, blood vessels, and nerves (vital organs)
(21) Large intestine (vessel organs)

mKhris.Pa then progresses in the:
(22) Blood (bodily constituents)
(23) Perspiration (excretion)
(24) Eyes (sense organs)
(25) Liver (vital organs)
(26) Gall bladder and small intestine (vessel organs)

Bad.Kan then progresses in the:
(27) Nutritional essence, muscles, fats, marrow, and regenerative fluids (bodily constituents)
(28) Feces and urine (excretions)
(29) Nose and tongue (sense organs)
(30) Lungs, spleen, and kidneys (vital organs)
(31) Stomach and urinary bladder (vessel organs)

Branch 6: The Period of Manifestation of Nyes.Pa

Stage of Life: [22]
(32) *Rlung* is the natural condition of the aged, when the overall physical energy is greatly reduced. The aged are more susceptible to *Rlung* disorders.
(33) *mKhris.Pa* is the optimal natural condition of adults, when the overall physical energy is at its peak, the individual is full of confidence and short-tempered. The adults are more susceptible to *mKhris.Pa* disorders.
(34) *Bad.Kan* is the natural condition of childhood, when the overall physical energy is just developing. The children are more susceptible to *Bad.Kan* disorders.

Climate and Locale:
(35) *Rlung* disorders thrive in cold and windy regions.
(36) *mKhris.Pa* disorders thrive in hot and dry regions.
(37) *Bad.Kan* disorders thrive in wet and humid regions.

Season and Daily Period:
(38) *Rlung* disorders increase during summer, especially in the evening and early morning.
(39) *mKhris.Pa* disorders increase during autumn, especially at noon and midnight.

(40) Bad.Kan disorders increase during spring, especially at dusk and dawn.

Branch 7: Disorders Leading to Terminal Conditions[23]

(41) Exhaustion of one's life span, karma, or merit.[24]

(42) The simultaneous combination of advanced hot and cold disorders. This causes the former to destroy the latter and vice versa and creates a destructive cycle. The treatments cannot effectively respond to the rapid shift of the opposing conditions needing immediate treatment.

(43) Identical application refers to the application of four-remedies[25] similar to either the hot or cold nature of the disorders. Therefore, instead of alleviating, it exacerbates the disorders, i.e., for a fever, sitting in the hot sun, taking a hot bath, taking warming foods and beverages, or medicines will all cause the fever to increase.

(44) Infliction of wounds caused by weapons (foreign bodies, bullets, etc.) to vulnerable points, organs, or life vessels (major blood vessels and nerves).

(45) A hot disorder that has gone beyond its treatment limit.

(46) A cold disorder that has fallen below its recovery limit.

(47) Exhaustion of bodily constituents due to any kind of emaciating or chronic wasting diseases, which reduces the patient's tolerance of the treatment.

(48) *Rlung* disorder that has gone beyond its treatment limit interrupts the life-supporting *Rlung*, called the wisdom *Rlung* (*Rlung dBu.Ma*, the *Rlung* of central channel). As a direct result, respiration comes to an end.

(49) The person will certainly die if the evil spirits have stolen the vital life force (*Bla*[26]). The evil spirits gain the opportunity when a person experiences great fear or a decline of the level of health, energies, or merit (positive karma).

Branch 8: Causes of Adverse Reactions[27]

Table 1.3.3: Causes of Adverse Reactions

Treated Disorder	Mistreatment	Result to Treated Disorder	Exacerbates
Rlung	Excess	Pacified	(50) *mKhris.Pa*
"	"	"	(51) *Bad.Kan*
"	Perverse	Not pacified	(52) *mKhris.Pa*
"	"	"	(53) *Bad.Kan*
mKhris.Pa	Excess	Pacified	(54) *Rlung*
"	"	"	(55) *Bad.Kan*
"	Perverse	Not pacified	(56) *Rlung*
"	"	"	(57) *Bad.Kan*
Bad.Kan	Excess	Pacified	(58) *Rlung*

"	"	"	(59) *mKhris.Pa*
"	Perverse	Not pacified	(60) *Rlung*
"	"	"	(61) *mKhris.Pa*

Branch 9: Summation

(62) **Cold**: *Rlung* and *Bad.Kan*, like water, are cool by nature.
(63) **Hot**: Blood and *mKhris.Pa*, like fire, are hot by nature.

Microorganisms and lymph systems are neutral by nature and can be either hot or cold depending on the predominance of the *Nyes.Pa*. One will thus understand all the basic concepts of the body and diseases from the enumeration of eighty-eight leaves. This concludes the third chapter, the basis of the normal and abnormal body from the Secret Oral Instruction's Tantra on the Eight Branches of the Essence of Nectar.

CHAPTER FOUR

DIAGNOSIS

Immediately following the teachings of chapter three, the sage Rig.Pa'i Ye.Shes spoke these words, "Oh great sage, listen. Each and entire categories of the diseases may be known from visual examination, touch, and interrogation." See the following Table 1.4.1 for number of trunks, branches, and leaves on the Root of Diagnosis. Refer to Figure 1.4.1, the Allegorical Tree of the Diagnosis.

Table 1.4.1: The Root of Diagnosis

Trunk No.	Branches	Leaves
1. Visual examination	2	6
2. Touch	3	3
3. Interrogation	3	29
Total	8	38

Trunk Number One

Trunk Number One represents the visual examination, and on it spreads the branches of tongue and urine examinations. On these branches, in turn, grow three and three leaves. A sequential explanation of each of these leaves follows.

Branch 1: Tongue
(1) **Rlung disorder**: Reddish, dry, and coarse
(2) **mKhris.Pa disorder**: Whitish-yellow with thick coating
(3) **Bad.Kan disorder**: Pale, dull, smooth, and moist with sticky coating

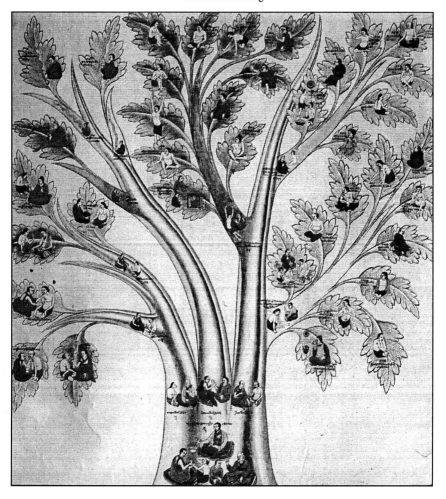

Figure 1.4.1: Allegorical Tree of the Diagnosis

Note: For more information, see Part Two, Secondary Diagnosis for Examining the Tongue.

Branch 2: Urine

(4) **Rlung disorder:**   Spring-water-like clear, bluish and thin with large bubbles when stirred

(5) **mKhris.Pa disorder:**   Reddish-yellow with lots of steam, foul odor, and quickly disappearing tiny bubbles when stirred

(6) **Bad.Kan** disorder: Whitish with light odor and steam, and saliva-like bubbles when stirred

Note: For more information, see Part Two, Diagnosis by Urine Examination.

Trunk Number Two

Trunk Number Two represents the pulse examination, and on it spreads the branches of *Rlung, mKhris.Pa,* and *Bad.Kan* disorders' pulse. On these branches, in turn, grow one, one, and one leaves. A sequential explanation of each of the leaves follows.

Branch 1: Rlung Disorder's Pulse
(7)   Thick-like sack distended by air that floats on the surface and is empty when pressed; there is a pause between pulse beats at indefinite (pulse) counts.

Branch 2: mKhris.Pa Disorder's Pulse
(8)   Fast, prominent, and does not halt when pressed, and is thin and taut like rolled horse tail.

Branch 3: Bad.Kan Disorder's Pulse
(9)   Unclear and deeply sunken, weak and slow

Note: For more information, see Part Two, Diagnosis by Pulse Examination.

Trunk Number Three

Trunk Number Three represents the interrogation, and on it spreads the branches of *Rlung, mKhris.Pa,* and *Bad.Kan* interrogation. On these branches, in turn, grow eleven, seven, and eleven leaves. A sequential explanation of each of these follows.

Branch 1: Interrogation for Rlung Disorder

Immediate Causes:
(10) Excessive intake of goat meat, pork, and tea, light and coarse powered foods and beverages, indulging in fasting, and exposure to cold wind.

Signs and Symptoms:
(11) Yawning and trembling
(12) Frequent stretching of limbs
(13) Cold chills

(14) Pain in hips, waist, and all the joints

(15) Uncertain moving pain

(16) Empty emesis

(17) Dullness of the eyes, sense organs

(18) Mentally becomes light, restless, and short-tempered

(19) Pain when hungry

Response:

(20) Responds well to the oily and nutritious foods and beverages, warm and tension-free lifestyle.

Branch 2: Interrogation for mKhris.Pa Disorder

Immediate Causes:

(21) Excessive intake of meat, one-year-old butter, seed oil, molasses, and alcohol, sharp and heat inducing foods and beverages, and excessive exposure to sun or fire.

Signs and Symptoms:

(22) Bitter taste in mouth

(23) Headache

(24) Rise of surface temperature

(25) Severe pain in upper body

(26) Pain, especially after food has been digested

Response:

(27) Responds well to the cooling powered foods, beverages, and lifestyle

Branch 3: Interrogation for Bad.Kan Disorder

Immediate Causes:

(28) Excessive intake of marmot meat, withered leaves, unripened fruits, and milk, heavy and greasy powered foods and beverages, and staying too long in damp places.

Signs and Symptoms:

(29) Loss of appetite

(30) Difficulty in digesting food

(31) Frequent vomiting

(32) Unclear perception of taste

(33) Distension of stomach

(34) Frequent belching

(35) Simultaneous heaviness of body and mind

(36) Feeling of coldness on surface as well as internal

(37) Discomfort after eating

Response:

(38) Responds well to warming powered foods, beverages, and lifestyle

Note: See Chapter Five, Methods of Healing for wholesome foods and beverages and behavioral pattern for *Rlung, mKhris.Pa,* and *Bad.Kan* disorders.

Thus, there are six leaves on visual examination, three on touch, and twenty-nine on interrogation. In total there are thirty-eight leaves on diagnosis. These will enable one to differentiate healthy and unhealthy as well as unmistakably ascertain each and every disease. That concludes the fourth chapter, the diagnosis from the Secret Oral Instruction's Tantra on the Eight Branches of the Essence of Nectar.

CHAPTER FIVE

METHODS OF HEALING

Immediately following the teachings of Chapter Four, the sage Rig.Pa'i Ye.Shes spoke these words, "Oh great sage, listen. The remedies for healing diseases are (explained here with the help of Figure 1.5.1, the Allegorical Tree consisting of): (1) diet, (2) behavioral pattern, (3) medicine, and (4) accessory therapy." See the Table 1.5.1 below for the number of trunks, branches, and leaves on the Root of Methods of Healing.

Table 1.5.1: The Root of the Methods of Healing

Trunk No.	Branches	Leaves
1. Diet	6	35
2. Behavior	3	6
3. Medicines	15	50
4. Accessory therapy	3	7
Total	27	98

Trunk Number One

Trunk Number One represents diet, and on it spreads the branches of wholesome foods for *Rlung* disorder, wholesome beverages for *Rlung* disorder, wholesome foods for *mKhris.Pa* disorder, wholesome beverages for *mKhris.Pa* disorder, wholesome foods for *Bad.Kan* disorder, and wholesome beverages for *Bad.Kan* disorder. On these branches, in turn, grow ten, four, nine, three, six, and three leaves. A sequential explanation of each of these leaves follows.

Branch 1: Wholesome Foods for Rlung Disorder

(1) Horse meat*[1]
(2) Donkey meat*
(3) Marmot meat*

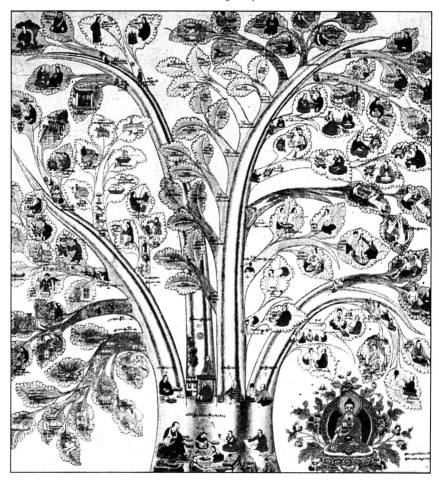

Figure 1.5.1: The Allegorical Tree of the Methods of Healing

(4)   One-year-old dry meat
(5)   *Sha.Chen* (Great meat)*[2]
(6)   Sesame oil, seed oil
(7)   One-year-old butter
(8)   Molasses
(9)   Garlic
(10) Onion

Branch 2: Wholesome Beverages for Rlung Disorder

(11) Warm milk
(12) *Zan.Chang*[3] made from Angelica sp. and Polygonatum cirrhifolium Royle

42

(13) Wine made from molasses as main ingredient
(14) Wine made from crushed bone as main ingredient

Branch 3: Wholesome Foods for mKhris.Pa Disorder

(15) Curd from cow's or goat's milk
(16) Buttermilk from cow's or goat's milk[4]
(17) Fresh butter
(18) Meat of a herbivorous animal*
(19) Goat meat
(20) *sKom.Po* (*rTol.Sha gSar.Pa*): Fresh meat of cross-bred offspring of *mDzo.Mo*[5] with ox or yak
(21) Thin noodles made from freshly pounded barley
(22) Noodles made from white dandelion (Taraxacum sp.)
(23) Noodles made from dandelion (Taraxacum officinale Web)

Branch 4: Wholesome Beverages for mKhris.Pa Disorder

(24) Tea[6] with no butter, milk, or salt or thin noodles made from *rTsam.Pa* (roasted barley flour) with no salt, meat, or fat
(25) Cool water from snow from a rocky mountain
(26) Boiled cold water

Branch 5: Wholesome Foods for Bad.Kan Disorder

(27) Mutton
(28) Wild yak meat*
(29) Carnivorous animal's meat*
(30) Fish
(31) Honey
(32) Warm dough made from *rTsam.Pa* (roasted barley flour) of one-year-old grain, grown in hot and dry areas with butter of sheep or *'Bri* (female yak)

Branch 6: Wholesome Beverages for Bad.Kan Disorder

(33) Curd and buttermilk from *'Bri*'s milk
(34) Concentrated old *Chang* (wine)
(35) Boiled hot water

Trunk Number Two

Trunk Number Two represents behavioral patterns, and on it spreads the branches of behavioral patterns for *Rlung* disorder, *mKhris.Pa* disorder, and *Bad.Kan* disorder.

On these branches, in turn, grow two, two, and two leaves. A sequential explanation of each of these leaves follows.

Branch 1: Behavioral Pattern for Rlung Disorder

(36) Abiding in a dim and warm place
(37) Enjoying the company of one's beloved while mentally relaxed and stress-free

Branch 2: Behavioral Pattern for mKhris.Pa Disorder

(38) Abiding by the river or lake, or cool place
(39) Abiding relaxed and restful

Branch 3: Behavioral Pattern for Bad.Kan Disorder

(40) Jogging, exercises, and exposure to sun
(41) Abiding in warm places and wearing warm clothes

Trunk Number Three

Trunk Number Three represents medicine, and on it spreads the branches of tastes of medicines for *Rlung* disorder and inherent qualities of medicines for *Rlung* disorder, fifteen branches. The branches numbers seven to twelve come in the category of pacification medicines, and thirteen to fifteen come in the category of cleansing medicines. See notes 9 and 10 of Part One, Chapter Two for explanation of pacification and cleansing medicines. On these branches grow fifty leaves. A sequential explanation of each of these leaves follows.

Branch 1: Tastes of Medicines for Rlung Disorder

(42) **Sweet** (*Bu.Ram*; molasses)
(43) **Sour** (*Chang.rGan*; old wine)
(44) **Salty** (*rGyam.Tsha*; sodium chloride)

Branch 2: Inherent Qualities of Medicines for Rlung Disorder

(45) **Oily** (*Ar.Nag*; Aquilaria agollocha Roxb.)
(46) **Heavy** (*Kha.Ru.Tsha*; black salt)
(47) **Smooth** (*Kan.Da Ka.Ri*; Rubus idaeopsis Focke.)

Branch 3: Tastes of Medicines for mKhris.Pa Disorder

(48) **Sweet** (*rGun.'Brum*; Vitis vinifera Wall)
(49) **Bitter** (*gSer.Me*; Herpetospermum pedunculosum)
(50) **Astringent** (*Tsan.Dan dKar.Po*; Santalum album Linn)

Branch 4: Inherent Qualities of Medicines for mKhris.Pa Disorder

(51) **Cool** (*Ga.Bur*; Cinnamomum camphora Nees)
(52) **Fluid** (*Dong.Ga*; Cassia fistula Linn.)
(53) **Blunt** (*Cu.Gang*; Bambusa textilis)

Branch 5: Tastes of Medicines for Bad.Kan Disorder

(54) **Hot** (*Na.Le.Sham*; Piper nigrum Linn.)
(55) **Sour** (*Se.'Bru*; Punica granatum Linn.)
(56) **Astringent** (*Ba.Ru*; Terminalia belerica)

Branch 6: Inherent Qualities of Medicines for Bad.Kan Disorder

(57) **Sharp** (*rGya.Tsha*; Rock salt)
(58) **Coarse** (*sTar.Bu*; Hippophae rhamnoides Linn.)
(59) **Light** (*Tsi.Tra.Ka*; Capsicum fructescens.)

Branch 7: Soups That Pacify Rlung Disorder

(60) Broth made from the nutritious bones (ankle, end of scapula where you can grasp (*Sog.Yu*), and sacral bones)
(61) Soup extracted from four nutritious foods (meat, butter, molasses, and old *Chang*)
(62) Broth made from three-year-old head of sheep, aged two years

Branch 8: Medicinal Butters That pacify Rlung Disorder

(63) Medicinal butter with *Dza'.Ti* (nutmeg) as its main ingredient.
(64) Medicinal butter with *sGog.sKya* (garlic) as its main ingredient.
(65) Medicinal butter with the three fruits *A.Ru* (Terminalia chebula), *Ba.Ru* (Terminalia belerica), and *sKyu.Ru* (Embelica officinalis) as its main ingredients.
(66) Medicinal butter with the five roots *Ba.sPru* (Withania somnifera), *gZe.Ma* (Tribulus terrestris Linn.), *lCa.Ba* (Angelica sp.), *Ra.mNye* (Polygonatum cirrhifolium Royle), and *Nye.Shing* (Asparagus racemosus) as its main ingredients.

(67) Medicinal butter with *sMan.Chen* (Aconitum balfouri Wall) as its main ingredient.

Branch 9: Decoctions That Pacify mKhris.Pa Disorder

(68) Decoction with *Ma.Nu* (Inula recemosa Hook) as its main ingredient
(69) Decoction with *sLe.Tres* (Tinospora cordifolia Miers) as its main ingredient
(70) Decoction with *Tig.Ta* (Swertia chirata) as its main ingredient
(71) Decoction with the three fruits Terminalia chebula, Terminalia belerica, and Emblica officinalis as its main ingredients

Branch 10: Medicinal Powders That Pacify mKhris.Pa Disorder

(72) Medicinal powder with *Ga.Bur* (Cinnamomum camphora) as its main ingredient

(73) Medicinal powder with *Tsan.Dan dKar.Po* (Santalum album Linn) as its main ingredient

(74) Medicinal powder with *Gur.Gum* (Carthamus tinctorius Linn) as its main ingredient

(75) Medicinal powder with *Cu.Gang* (Bambusa textilis) as its main ingredient

Branch 11: Medicinal Pills That Pacify Bad.Kan Disorder

(76) Medicinal pill with *sMan.Chen* (Aconitum balfouri Wall) as its main ingredient

(77) Medicinal pill with *Tsha* (Sodium chloride), *Kha.Ru.Tsha* (black salt), and *rGyam.Tsha* (rock salt), various salts as its main ingredients.

Branch 12: Medicinal Powders That Pacify Bad.Kan Disorder

(78) Medicinal powder with *Se.'Bru* (Punica granatum Linn) as its main ingredient.

(79) Medicinal powder with *Da.Li* (Rhododendron aff. cephalantum) as its main ingredient.

(80) Medicinal powder whose compound is known as *sNod.sByin rGod.Ma.Kha* (the mouth of a *yaksha*, harmful spirit),[6] a powerful heat-inducing medicine with *Ka.Ran.Za* (Caesalpinia sepiaria) as its main ingredient.

(81) Medicinal powder with calcinated *Tsha* (salt) as its main ingredient.

(82) Medicinal powder with calcinated *Cong.Zhi* (calcite) as its main ingredient.

Branch 13: Suppositories for Rlung Disorder

(83) *sLe.'Jam*: A mild enema, which involves the procedure of inserting medi-

cine through the anal canal to evacuate the *Rlung* disorders from the intestinal region.

(84) **bKru.'Jam**: A moderate enema consisting of *sLe.'Jam* plus another formula. It is then inserted through the anal canal to the patient, who lies on his/her back while physician gently taps the soles of the feet to evacuate the *Rlung* and *mKhris.Pa* combined disorders from the intestinal region.

(85) **bKru.Ma sLen**: A strong enema with another additional formula added to *bKru.'Jam*. It is then inserted through the anal canal to the patient. The physician holds patient by the feet and shakes up and down to evacuate the *Rlung* and *Bad.Kan* combined disorder from the intestinal region.

Branch 14: Purgatives for mKhris.Pa Disorder

(86) **sPyi.bShal** (General purgative): An initial preparation as part of the general purgative consists of taking bath with mixture of *mKhan.Pa* (Artemisia sp.), *sBang.Ma* (residue of Chang), and warm water. It is followed by whole body massage (except lower abdomen) by fresh butter or sesame seed oil depending on hot or cold disorders, respectively.

(87) **sGos.bShal** (Specific purgative): After taking the purgative specifically for one's illness the patient rinses his/her mouth.

(88) **Drag.bShal** (Drastic purgative): If vomiting is induced, it is suppressed by pressing the patient by the shoulders, pulling his/her hair from the crown of the head, and sprinkling cold water on face.

(89) **'Jam.bShal** (Smooth purgative): After giving it, a hot compress is put on the patient's abdomen.

Branch 15: Emetics for Bad.Kan Disorder

(90) **Drag.sKyug** (Drastic emetic): After taking the emetic, the patient is advised to bend his/her knees up to the abdomen and sit in a squatting posture.

(91) **'Jam.sKyug** (Smooth emetic): The patient is advised to cover him/herself with warm clothes and then sit in a squatting posture.

Trunk Number Four

Trunk Number Four represents accessory therapy, and on it spreads the branches of therapy for *Rlung* disorder, *mKhris.Pa* disorder, and *Bad.Kan* disorder. On these branches, in turn, grow two, three, and two leaves. A sequential explanation of each of these leaves follows.

Branch 1: Therapy for Rlung Disorder

(92) **bsKu.mNye**: Massage with Til.Mar (Sesamum indicum Linn.), oil.

(93) **Hor.Gyi Me.bTsa'**: *Go.sNyod* (Carum carvi Linn.) is put in cloth, immersed in warm sesamum oil, and used as a compress at various *Rlung* points.

Branch 2: Therapy for mKhris.Pa Disorder

(94) **rNgul dByung.Ba**: To sweat, a patient is kept under thick coverings.
(95) **gTar.Ga**: Blood is let from various points of veins.
(96) **Chu.Yi 'Phrul.'Khor**: Patient is advised to have a cold shower or stay under a waterfall.

Branch 3: Therapy for Bad.Kan Disorder

(97) **Dugs**: A hot compress is given on the abdomen, by heated salt wrapped in cloth.
(98) **Me.bTsa'**: Moxibustion at specific points on the abdomen and body joints.

Thus, there are ninety-eight methods of healing. If a physician applies these with full attention, care, and diligence, the patient will soon be freed from the mire of diseases. This concludes the fifth chapter, the methods of healing from the Secret Oral Instruction's Tantra on the Eight Branches of the Essence of Nectar.

CHAPTER SIX

THE SUMMARY OF ROOT TANTRA

Immediately following the teachings of Chapter Five, once again, the sage *Rig.Pa'i Ye.Shes* spoke these words, "Oh great sage, listen. Based on Allegorical Tree, the preceding three chapters of Root Tantra are enumerated here in brief. The three chapters (roots) are: (1) the basis of the normal and abnormal body, (2) diagnosis, and (3) methods of healing. On these roots, grow nine trunks. They are: (1) normal and (2) abnormal body, (3) the visual, (4) touch, (5) interrogation, (6) diet, (7) behavioral pattern, (8) medicine, and (9) accessory therapy."

On these trunks spread out forty-seven branches. The branches on the normal body (first trunk) are: (1) fifteen afflictions, (2) seven bodily constituents, and (3) three excretions.

The branches on the abnormal body (second trunk) are: (4) the primary causes, (5) the immediate causes, (6) general passages, (7) general locations, (8) the progression of *Nyes.Pa*, (9) period of manifestation of *Nyes.Pa*, (10) terminal conditions, (11) adverse reactions, and (12) summation.

The branches on the visual examination (third trunk) are: (13) tongue and (14) urine. The branches on the touch examination (fourth trunk) are: (15) the *Rlung* disorder's pulse, (16) *mKhris.Pa* disorder's pulse, and (17) *Bad.Kan* disorder's pulse. The branches on the interrogation (fifth trunk) are: (18) the interrogation for *Rlung* disorder, (19) interrogation for *mKhris.Pa* disorder, and (20) interrogation for *Bad.Kan* disorder.

The branches on the diet (sixth trunk) are: (21) foods for *Rlung* disorder, (22) beverages for *Rlung* disorder, (23) foods for *mKhris.Pa* disorder, (24) beverages for *mKhris.Pa* disorder, (25) foods for *Bad.Kan* disorder, and (26) beverages for *Bad.Kan* disorder. The branches on the behavioral pattern (seventh trunk) are: (27) behavioral pattern for *Rlung* disorder, (28) behavioral pattern for *mKhris.Pa* disorder, and (29) behavioral pattern for *Bad.Kan* disorder.

The branches on the tastes and inherent qualities of medicines (eighth trunk) are: (30) tastes of medicines for *Rlung* disorder, (31) qualities of medicines for *Rlung* disorder, (32) tastes for *mKhris.Pa* disorder, (33) qualities for *mKhris.Pa* disorder, (34) tastes for *Bad.Kan* disorder, and (35) qualities for *Bad.Kan* disorder. The branches on the pacification medicine are: (36) soups for *Rlung* disorder, (37) medicinal butters for *Rlung* disorder, (38) decoctions for *mKhris.Pa* disorder, (39) powdered medicines for *mKhris.Pa* disorder, (40) medicinal pills for *Bad.Kan* disorder, (41) medicinal powders for *Bad.Kan* disorder, (42) suppositories for *Rlung* disorder, (43) purgatives for *mKhris.Pa* disorder, and (44) emetics for *Bad.Kan* disorder.

The branches on the accessory therapy (ninth trunk) are: (45) therapy for *Rlung* disorder, (46) therapy for *mKhris.Pa* disorder, and (47) therapy for *Bad.Kan* disorder.

The enumeration of the number of leaves developed on these forty-seven branches are: twenty-five leaves on the first (normal body) trunk, sixty-three leaves on the second (abnormal body) trunk, six leaves on the third (visual examination) trunk, three leaves on the fourth (touch) trunk, and twenty-nine leaves on the fifth (interrogation) trunk.

On the sixth (diet) trunk, there are thirty-five leaves. They are: fourteen leaves of diet for *Rlung* disorder, twelve leaves of diet for *mKhris.Pa* disorder, and nine leaves of diet for *Bad.Kan* disorder. There are six leaves on the seventh (behavioral pattern) trunk. On the eighth (medicine) trunk, there are fifty leaves. They are: nine leaves on tastes of medicine, nine leaves on inherent qualities of medicine, three leaves on soup, five leaves on medicinal butter, four leaves on decoction, four leaves on medicinal powder, two leaves on pills, five leaves on medicinal powder, and nine leaves on unsurpassed (cleansing works). On the ninth (accessory therapy) trunk, there are seven leaves.

Thus, there are 88 leaves for the basis of the normal and abnormal body, 38 leaves for diagnosis, and 98 leaves for methods of healing. In all there develops 224 leaves on these 47 branches.

On the first trunk (normal body) blossom the flowers of freedom from disease and long life and matures the fruits of high spiritual life, wealth, and happiness. Though these fruits are said to be attained by persons with normal health, it also implies something to a physician, whose job it is to keep others free of diseases.

The chapters are expounded, based on Ashoka tree's (Tib: *Mya.Ngan Med.Pa'i lJon.Shing*; Eng: Saraca Indica), root, and trunk, etc. The Ashoka tree is used in all ancient Tibetan medical texts to illustrate the precise meaning and confer a comprehensive knowledge of the Science of Healing. *Ashoka* is comprised of two words: a which means "not" and *shoka* which means "grief" thus, the Ashoka is used to represent the healthy body and mind. This essence of (subsequent three tantras, namely explanatory, oral instruction's, and last tantra) Root Tantra will be understood and applied by some sharp intellects whereas persons with poor intellect will not understand this. Those who desire further research and to study more elaborate and detailed text should look for subsequent tantras as well as other great treatises on the medical system.

After expounding the First Tantra, the sage *Rig.Pa'i Ye.Shes* dissolved back into the heart of the King of Physicians. This concludes the sixth chapter, the summary of Root Tantra as well as treatise of Root Tantra from the Secret Oral Instruction's Tantra on the Eight Branches of the Essence of Nectar.

Part Two
Diagnosis

CHAPTER ONE

DIAGNOSIS BY PULSE EXAMINATION

The practices of Tibetan pulse and urine examinations appear simple, yet they are very complex diagnostic techniques. An in-depth study of the two subjects is essential for building the skills necessary for a correct diagnosis.

For instance, the pulse is like a messenger who gives the messages from the patient's abnormal site to a physician. The messages, like a *weak* or *strong* pulse beat, are transmitted to the radial artery by *Rlung*. *Rlung* is an energy that governs the functions of the nervous system, respiration, cardiovascular system, and many other things. Messages are picked up at the radial artery by a physician's index, middle, and ring fingers of both hands.

Under Tibetan medical study, pulse examination is considered diagnosis by touch. Diagnosis by touch refers to the physician's feeling with his or her hand at various parts or vital points of the patient's body. It will help him or her to identify the degree of body temperature and to confirm the growth of external cysts or abnormalities. Sensitivity of certain points in the body gives good clues to correlate with other related major or minor problems and can result in a more accurate diagnosis.

Pulse examination is explained in the thirteen sections in the Last Tantra of the *rGyud.bZhi*, and their explanation follows in order.

Prerequisite Conditions

The patient should observe certain preliminary dietary and lifestyle restrictions one day prior to the day of the actual pulse examination so that no disturbances are caused to the actual state of his or her illness. The patient should refrain from the following things to avoid altering pulse characteristics:

Meat and alcohol (such as lamb, yak meat, and poultry, considered warming foods and drinks, to avoid a mistaken diagnosis of a hot disorder.
Excessive strong tea, coffee, goat meat, and pork (light and coarse powered foods and drinks), to avoid a mistaken diagnosis of a *Rlung* disorder.

Refrigerated, stale foods and unripened fruits (cooling and difficult to digest), to avoid a mistaken diagnosis of a *Bad.Kan* disorder.

Excessive eating and drinking: to avoid a mistaken diagnosis of a hot disorder due to a high and taut pulse beat.

Intense hunger and fasting: to avoid a mistaken diagnosis of a cold disorder due to a low and weak pulse beat.

Too much talking, sex, sleepless nights, and activities causing physical and mental stress, to avoid a mistaken diagnosis of a *Rlung* disorder.

The doctor should be of good health and have clear sensual and mental perceptions and should pay full attention to the patient's problem. Whether or not the doctor can fully concentrate depends on the freshness of his or her body and mind. Therefore, the doctor should refrain from excessive:

> **sleepless nights,**
> **alcohol,**
> **sex,**
> **talking, and**
> **physical and mental stress.**

During the examination, the doctor's respiration, body temperature, and pulse beat should also be normal. In order to prevent misdiagnosis, the patient should be relaxed; the pulse should not be read immediately after he or she has engaged in physical exertion or sat in the sun, both of which would effect respiration, body temperature, and pulse.

Time of Pulse Examination

The best time to read the pulse is in the morning when the lines on the palms are clearly visible. That is also a time when the external and internal hot and cold energies are at an equal level. Though it is almost impossible to put into practice, the text explains that the doctor should be alert for the following six conditions, which, if present, may affect a misdiagnosis.

- The rise of warmth in a patient's body (which may cause a mistaken diagnosis of a blood and *mKhris.Pa* disorder if the patient is examined during the day).
- The predominance of cold in the night (which may cause a mistaken diagnosis of a cold disorder).
- The patient has not excessively exhaled his or her warm air by either reciting mantras or reading scriptures, etc.
- The patient has not inhaled cold air from outside.
- The patient has not moved or risen from bed.

- The patient has either over or under-indulged in food and drink.

Site of Pulse Examination

Under this topic, examining the pulse at the radial artery, the near death pulse, and vital life force pulse are explained in order.

Examining the Pulse at the Radial Artery

The best site for reading the pulse is at the radial artery. The physician places his or her index, middle, and ring fingers of the right and left hand on the radial artery of the patient's left and right wrist respectively, measuring the length of the patient's distal phalanx of the thumb from the first crease of the wrist. The physician's fingers should be neither too close nor too far apart. (Refer to Figure 2.1.3 to see the correct method of finger placement on the patient's wrist.)

The Near Death Pulse

The near death pulse is read at the patient's dorsalis pedis artery (*Bol.Gong 'Phar.rTsa 'Am Bol.Gong 'Gul.rTsa Nag.Po*) of both feet. This is examined because the energies and the elements withdraw gradually from the feet toward the heart, indicated by loss of heat from there. Figure 2.1.1 below shows the near death pulse.

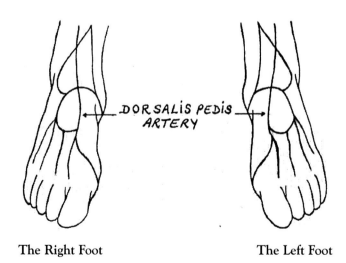

| The Right Foot | The Left Foot |

Figure 2.1.1: The Near Death Pulse

Vital Life Force (*Bla*) Pulse

The vital life force (*Bla*) pulse is read on the ulnar artery on the inside of the wrist. *Bla* is a force that supports in sustaining a life; therefore, *Bla* is also considered the mother of life. The explanation also appears at the end of this chapter, the vital Life Force (*Bla*) Pulse. Figure 2.1.2 below shows the vital life force pulse.

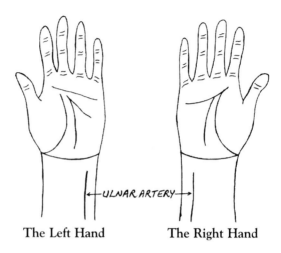

The Left Hand   The Right Hand

Figure 2.1.2: The Vital Life Force Pulse

Amount of pressure

The amount of pressure applied by each of the physician's fingers is as follows:
- The index fingers (*Tshon*) should be pressed lightly to feel the skin.
- The middle fingers (*Kan*) should be pressed moderately to feel flesh.
- The ring fingers (*Chag*) should be pressed strongly to feel bone.

The radial artery deepens as it goes from wrist to elbow, and hence it becomes necessary to feel it in this way.

Methods of Pulse Examination

The physician's fingers should be smooth, flexible, sensitive, and warm. The left wrist of a male patient is examined first, whereas the right wrist is examined first for a female. Then the opposite wrists are examined.

Placement of organs beneath the fingers is shown in Figure 2.1.3, which denotes the finger placement for taking the pulse of a man. Note that for females the organs beneath the index fingers are reversed from those for males (i. e., the heart and small intestine are read by the physician's left hand, the lungs and large intestine by the right), while the organs beneath the other fingers are the same.

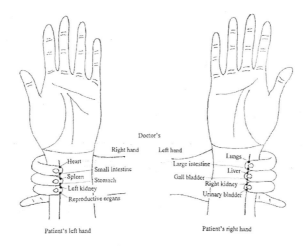

Doctor's
Right hand   Left hand
Heart   Lungs
          Small intestine   Large intestine   Liver
Spleen   Stomach   Gall bladder
Left kidney   Right kidney
          Reproductive organs   Urinary bladder

Patient's left hand   Patient's right hand

Figure 2.1.3: Method of Finger Placement

This differentiation is made because the channels through which mental consciousness moves in the heart are closer to the left side for males and to the right side for females. The secret mantra in ancient Buddhist tantra text explains that the channels through which mental consciousness moves in the tip of the heart are pointed toward the left channel (Skt: *Lalana*; Tib: *rKyang.Ma*)[1] for males and the right (Skt: *Rasana*; Tib: *Ro.Ma*)[2] for females.

The conditions of the upper, middle, and lower parts of the body are also examined by the index, middle, and ring fingers, respectively. Refer to 2.1.4, which shows a close-up view of the exact position of finger placement.

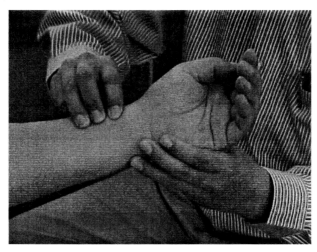

Figure 2.1.4: A Close-Up View of the Exact Position of Finger Placement

The primary constituents of an offspring depend on its father's sperm and mother's ovum. The lifestyle, eating, and drinking habits of the mother while pregnant also play a great role in determining her offspring's constitutional pulse and basic nature or attitude toward life. Note that the constitutional pulses *Male* and *Female* do not correspond to the person's gender but to the pulse characteristics.

Male pulse (Pho.rTsa): Thick and bulky pulse beat that corresponds partly to *Rlung* disorder's pulse.

Female pulse (Mo.rTsa): Thin and fast pulse beat that corresponds partly to a *mKhris.Pa* disorder's pulse.

Neuter pulse (Byang.Chub Sems.rTsa): Long in continuum, smooth, and flexible pulse beat that corresponds partly to a *Bad.Kan* disorder's pulse.

If for some reason the physician is unable to identify the constitutional pulse, he or she must ask the patient, since the male and female pulse can be mistaken for a hot disorder and the neuter pulse for a cold disorder.

- A thick and bulky male pulse can be mistaken for a hot disorder's strong and overflowing beat.
- A thin and fast female pulse can be mistaken for a hot disorder's taut and fast beat.
- A long in continuum, smooth, and flexible pulse beat can be mistaken for a cold disorder's slow, weak, and loose beat.

Although most non-Tibetans do not know their constitutional pulse type, some Tibetans are familiar with this concept or may have acquired the information from a previous diagnostic examination.

Once the constitutional pulse has been correctly identified, the physician is then able to classify the diseases into hot and cold categories. Table 2.1.1 illustrates the use of the constitutional pulse for diagnosis.

Table 2.1.1: Pulse Type and Interpretations

Pulse Type	Possessor	Interpretations
Male	Woman	More sons than daughters
Female	Man	Long life
Male	Both wife & husband	Most probably more male offspring

Female	”	Most probably more female offspring
Neutral	”	Will have long life, rarely fall ill and be loved by superiors; however, inferior people will consistently try to harm them, close relatives may become enemies and their lineage will come to an end
Male Neutral	Husband Wife	Only one son
Female Neutral	Wife Husband	Only one daughter

Seasonal Pulse

Under this topic, the mother/son and friend/foe relationships, solar and lunar influence on seasonal pulse, and influence of seasons on seasonal pulse are explained in order.

Mother/Son and Friend/Foe Relationships

The influence of cosmo-physical elements (*'Byung.Ba*) on the pulse is revealed primarily through changing seasonal variations due to solar-lunar effects on the environment. Before we examine these influences, it is first necessary to understand the relationships among the cosmo-physical elements (*'Byung.Ba*) themselves. These are revealed by the mother/son and friend/foe relationships in Figure 2.1.5, as well as their pulse nature and prognostication as illustrated in Table 2.1.2.

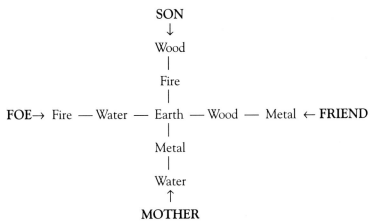

SON
↓
Wood
|
Fire
|
FOE→ Fire — Water — Earth — Wood — Metal ← **FRIEND**
|
Metal
|
Water
↑
MOTHER
Figure 2.1.5: Mother/Son & Friend/Foe Relationships

- The son of Wood is Fire, the son of Fire is Earth, the son of Earth is Metal, the son of Metal is Water, and the son of Water is Wood.
- The mother of Water is Metal, the mother of Metal is Earth, the mother of Earth is Fire, the mother of Fire is Wood, and the mother of Wood is Water.
- The foe of Fire is Water, the foe of Water is Earth, the foe of Earth is Wood, etc.
- The friend of Metal is Wood, the friend of Wood is Earth, the friend of Earth is Water, etc.

Table 2.1.2: Mother/Son and Friend/Foe Pulse Nature and Prognostication

Pulse Nature	Prognostication
Mother and Seasonal Pulse	The best of everything will be showered upon the person.
Son pulse	The individual will be very powerful.
Friend pulse	The individual will be wealthy, have good luck, and meet sincere friends.
Foe pulse	The individual will meet with enemies or be stricken with terminal disease.

Now let us study the above table in more detail. Suppose an individual is having his or her pulse prognosticated in spring, when the strength of the Wood element is at its peak and the energies within the liver/gall bladder are at their optimum level. During this season, if the seasonal pulse beat, i.e., the thin and taut pulse of Wood, and the smooth and slow pulse beat of Water (which is the mother of Wood), are both predominant, this signifies that the best of everything will be showered upon that individual.

Whichever of these pulses (the son, friend, or foe pulses) is predominant at their respective site, the prognostication is as indicated in the above chart. The application of this method is similar for summer, autumn, winter, and during the remaining eighteen days of each season when the Earth element predominates. Refer to Tables 2.1.3 and 2.1.4 for their application.

Solar and Lunar Influence on Seasonal Pulse

There are three main subtle energy channels in our body. They are *Ro.Ma*, *rKyang.Ma*, and *dBu.Ma*[3]. The *rKyang.Ma* channel is influenced by the Moon (Earth and Water elements), the *Ro.Ma* by the Sun (Fire element), and the *dBu.Ma* by neutral energy (Air element). The element Space is all-pervasive.

During the night the influence of lunar energy is stronger, and for this reason the pulse beat is normally slower and weaker. Likewise, the influence of solar energy is stronger during the day and the pulse beat is faster and stronger. Because of this, the better time to examine the pulse is when these two opposing influences are in a dynamic state of equilibrium—this occurs just at the break of dawn, when the quality of light allows one to see clearly the lines of one's palm.

Influence of Seasons on Seasonal Pulse

The traditional Tibetan astrological calendar has 360 days and is divided into four seasons—spring, summer, autumn, and winter. Each season consists of three months and each month equals thirty days. In pulse reading, each season is divided into two parts. The first seventy-two days of spring, summer, autumn, and winter are predominantly influenced by the elements Wood, Fire, Metal, and Water, respectively. The remaining eighteen days of each season are predominantly influenced by the Earth element. This is clarified in Table 2.1.3 below, which also shows the correspondence of season/element to body organs.

Table 2.1.3: Seasonal Influence on the Vital and Vessel Organs

Season	Months	Days	Element	Organs
Spring	1,2,3	72	Wood	liver/gall bladder
		18	Earth	spleen/stomach
Summer	4,5,6	72	Fire	heart/small intestine
		18	Earth	spleen/stomach
Autumn	7,8,9	72	Metal	lungs/large intestine
		18	Earth	spleen/stomach
Winter	10,11,12	72	Water	right kidney/urinary bladder, left kidney/ reproductive organs
		18	Earth	spleen/stomach

The influence of the Wood element is stronger on the liver and gall bladder pulse during the first seventy-two days of spring. Similarly, the heart and small intestine pulses are stronger during the first seventy-two days of summer; the lungs and large intestine pulses are stronger during the first seventy-two days of autumn; and the kidneys and urinary bladder and reproductive organ pulses are stronger during the first seventy-two days of winter. The influence of the Earth element is stronger on the spleen and stomach pulse during the remaining eighteen days of each season.

It is imperative for the physician to know the exact month and day of the season while checking a pulse in order to give a precise diagnosis. For instance, if a physician is not aware that he is checking the pulse during spring, then the stronger liver and gall bladder pulsations may be diagnosed as an ailment. See Table 2.1.4 below for the correlation of seasons, elements, and pulse characteristics. It is for this reason that the *rGyud.bZhi* gives an elaborate explanation of how a physician can identify the seasons through the observation of stars, bird migration, the growth cycles of trees and plants, and by use of the Tibetan Almanac.

Table 2.1.4: Seasons, Elements, and Pulse Characteristics

Season	Element	Pulse characteristics
Spring	Wood	thin and taut
Summer	Fire	thick and long in continuum
Autumn	Metal	coarse and short in continuum
Winter	Water	smooth and slow
remaining eighteen days of each season	Earth	smooth and short in continuum

The Seven Wondrous Pulse Examination

A very talented, experienced, and highly developed physician with insight acquired through meditation and religious practices related to medicine is able to foretell the issues and relations listed below. An experienced physician who is well-versed in these topics may also foretell these issues through elemental calculation. The seven wondrous pulse readings can be done only when the person making the inquiry (i.e., the one whose pulse is being examined) is free from any disorders. The seven wondrous pulses are:

- Family welfare pulse
- Arrival of guest pulse
- Harm from enemy pulse
- Friend or wealth pulse
- Evil spirits pulse
- Substitution pulse
- Pregnancy pulse

Because these topics are very complex, I shall focus only on the Substitutional and Pregnancy pulses.

The Substitutional Pulse

The substitutional pulse involves the assessment of the condition of an individual who is not within easy reach of the physician. To do this, the physician examines the pulse of a close friend or relative of the patient. For instance, a physician may examine a son or daughter's pulse in order to determine the health condition of a father or mother who is sick and not able to be examined directly. Using the techniques mentioned in the previous section, *Seasonal Pulse*, a physician can give a prognosis about the possibility of helping the father/mother/son/daughter. The ancient text explains four ways to use this technique.

(a) Examining the child's pulse when the parent is sick:
Regardless of seasons, if the son/daughter's Wood/Liver pulse is beating thin and taut, it means that the father/mother can be healed, whereas a missing beat implies a death. In terms of elemental calculations, if the Mother of the Seasonal pulse is beating properly, the patient can still be saved. If this pulse is missing, it is an indication of death. The principle of this practice is the same to all in this subsection.

(b) Examining the parent's pulse when the child is sick:
Regardless of seasons, if the father/mother's Fire/Heart pulse is beating thick and long in continuum, it indicates that the son/daughter can be healed, whereas a missing beat forecasts a death. In terms of elemental calculations, if the Son of the Seasonal pulse is beating properly, then the patient can still be saved. If this pulse is missing, it indicates that the patient will die.

(c) Examining the wife's pulse when the husband is sick:
Regardless of seasons, if the wife's Wood/Liver pulse is beating thin and taut, the husband can be healed, whereas the absence of this pulse indicates death. In terms of elemental calculations, if the Friend of the Seasonal pulse is beating properly, the husband will get better, whereas the absence of this pulse forecasts death.

(d) Examining the husband's pulse when the wife is sick:
Regardless of seasons, if the husband's Water/Kidney pulse is beating slowly and smoothly, the wife can be healed, whereas the absence of this pulse indicates death. In terms of elemental calculations, if the Enemy of the Seasonal pulse is beating properly, the wife will get better, whereas the absence of this pulse indicates death.

Pregnancy Pulse:

Though the pulse of both the patient with blood disorder and the pregnant woman beats with a protruding and rolling force, the pregnant woman's pulse beats stronger and faster. This is due to an ongoing demand for more blood due to the pregnancy, as well as the blood's activity in the woman's womb for the development of the fetus.

With respect to offspring, if the pulse beat of the right kidney is stronger and overflowing, the offspring will be male, and if the pulse beat of the left kidney is stronger and overflowing, the offspring will be female. The reason behind this difference is due to the position of the male and female fetus in the right and left side of the mother's womb.

In terms of elemental calculations, if the pregnant woman is being examined during the second Tibetan month (spring), the Son of the Seasonal pulse (i.e., the Fire/Heart pulse) becomes the basis from which to find that element's Mother and Son. The Son (Fire/Heart pulse) and the Seasonal pulse (Spring, Wood/Liver pulse) in turn are considered the pulse of the offspring and the pregnant woman. If the Mother (Wood/Liver) or Son's (Earth/Spleen) pulses beat at the site of the Fire/Heart pulse, the child will be easy to nurse after the delivery and will rarely fall ill. If the Enemy (Water/Kidneys) pulse beats at the site of the Fire/Heart pulse, the prognosis would be one of the following:

- The mother will die.
- The mother will experience a great pain during the delivery.
- The child will be difficult to nurse.
- If the child lives, he/she will grow up as an enemy to the mother.

Note: The pregnant woman's pulse can also be mistaken for a hot disorder's rolling and firm beat.

Healthy and Unhealthy Pulse Rate

Under this topic, the pulse rate of an adult, a child, a baby, and a healthy pulse beat are explained in order.

An Adult's Pulse Rate
If an adult's pulse beats five times during one respiratory count (i.e., one exhalation and inhalation) of the physician and remains so for fifteen of the physician's respiratory counts (one minute), he or she is considered healthy.

A Child's Pulse Rate
Likewise, for children, six beats during one respiratory count of the physician, is considered normal. That means, for physician's fifteen respiratory counts, the pulse beats will be ninety.

A Baby's Pulse Rate
For babies, eight beats during one respiratory count of the physician is normal. In

the physician's fifteen respiratory counts, the pulse beat will be one hundred and twenty. However, for children under eight years of age, instead of examining the pulse at the radial artery, their pulse is examined at the back of the ears. This is done due to the overall energies and strength of the child. Because the child is still growing, it is hard to differentiate the different pulse beats at the radial arteries.

Current practice for the duration of pulse examination is fifteen of the physician's respiratory counts. The duration the ancient text says to use is 100 of the physician's respiratory counts.

A Healthy Pulse Beat

A healthy pulse beat is devoid of following alternating beats:
- Strong and weak
- Thin at upper and thick at lower site
- Fast and slow
- Sunken and superficial
- Halts and pulls when it is supposed to be simply halting
- Taut and loose

If the pulse beat count is more or less than those mentioned above, the diagnosis is made as a hot or cold disorder, respectively. However, it is also normal for some people to have a slightly higher or lower pulse rate.

Unhealthy Pulse

Under this topic, general pulse beat, forty-seven specific pulse beats, ten additional pulse beats, and four critical points for determining the hot and cold disorders are explained.

General Pulse Beats

Under this subtopic, the six general pulse characteristics of hot and cold disorders, the six hot pulse beats and their associated disorders, and determining the severity of hot disorders from pulse characteristics, nine total subjects are explained.

(a) The six general pulse characteristics of hot and cold disorders:

Hot Disorder	Cold Disorder
(1) Strong (*Drag*)	Weak (*Zhan*)
(2) Overflowing (*rGyas*)	Sunken (*Bying*)
(3) Rolling (*'Dril*)	Declining (*Gud*)
(4) Fast (*mGyogs*)	Slow (*'Bul*)

(5) Taut (*Grims*)   Loose (*Lhod*)
(6) Firm (*mKhrang*)   Empty (*sTong*)

(b) The six hot pulse beats and their associated disorders:

Strong: High and disturbed fever
Overflowing (thick and high): *Rlung* and blood disturbances[4] and hot caused *Bad.Kan sMug.Po*[5]
Rolling: Blood disturbances and blood tumor
Fast: Acute infections and meat poisoning
Taut: *mKhris.Pa* and fever combined disorder and chronic fever
Firm: Septic wounds

(c) Determining the severity of hot disorders from pulse characteristics:
The appearance of:

- One or two pulse characteristics from the hot category above indicate a low fever
- Three or four pulse characteristics from the hot category above indicate a great fever
- Five or all six pulse characteristics from the hot category above indicate supreme or extreme fever

(d) Determining the severity of hot disorders from pulse rate:
The appearance of:

- Six beats within the physician's one respiratory count indicates a low fever
- Seven beats within the physician's one respiratory count indicates a great fever
- Eight beats within the physician's one respiratory count indicates a supreme or extreme fever
- Nine beats within the physician's one respiratory count indicates the fever has gone beyond its treatment limit

(e) Determining the Fresh And Chronic Hot Disorders:

Fresh Hot Disorders
dPang mTho.Ba: A pulse beat at the upper level (superficial) of the artery indicates a fresh disturbed fever. The strong and overflowing pulses (listed in the six general pulses above) beat at the upper level.

Grangs Mang.Ba:	A pulse rate greater than those previously mentioned (healthy and unhealthy pulse rates) indicates influenza. The rolling and fast pulses (listed in the six general pulses above) beat faster.

Chronic Hot Disorder

sNyugs.Kyi Tsha.Ba:	Sunken yet fast and short in continuum is an indication of chronic fever. The taut and firm pulses (listed in the six general pulses above) beats at the lower level of the arteries.

(f) The six cold pulse beats and their associated disorders:

Weak:	Tumor caused by cold disorder
Sunken:	Second and last stage edema
Declining:	First stage edema or anemia
Slow:	Cold lymph disorder[6] and pale *Bad.Kan* disorder[7]
Loose:	Cold tumor[8]
Empty:	*Rlung* disorders

(g) Determining the severity of cold disorders from pulse characteristics:
The appearance of:

- One or two pulse characteristics from the cold category above indicate a cold disorder
- Three or four pulse characteristics from the cold category above indicate a great cold disorder
- Five or all six pulse characteristics from the cold category above indicate supreme or extreme cold disorder

(h) Determining the severity of cold disorders from pulse rate:
The appearance of:

- Four beats within the physician's one respiratory count indicates mild cold disorder
- Three beats within the physician's one respiratory count indicates great cold disorder
- Two beats within the physician's one respiratory count indicates supreme cold disorder
- One beat in physician's one respiratory count indicates the cold has fallen below its treatment limit

(i) Determining the fresh and chronic cold disorders:

Fresh Cold Disorder
sNyugs.Grang:

> Pulse beats that are sunken yet are slow and long in continuum indicate a fresh cold disorder.

Chronic Cold Disorder
Grangs Nyung.Ba:

> Pulse rates less than those mentioned under healthy and unhealthy pulses indicate a chronic cold disorder.

dPang mTho.Ba:

> Pulse with low pulse rate that beats at the upper level (superficial) of the artery indicate a very chronic cold disorder.

In general, a hot disease is associated with *mKhris.Pa* and a cold disease with *Bad.Kan*. *Rlung* is neutral, and depending on the former two energies, it can be either hot or cold.

Forty-Seven Specific Pulse Beats

Under this subtopic, eleven general pulse beats (some are exceptions here), seven contagious fevers pulses, six temporal pulse beats, and seven hot disorders associated to the site are explained; they all come into the category of hot disorders. Also the six internal cold disorders, two secondary cold disorders, two secondary hot disorders (exceptions here), and clearing the six misconceptions are explained; they all come into the category of cold disorders.

(a) Eleven general pulse beats

(1) *Rlung* disorder:

> The pulse is thick, like a sack distended by air, floats on the surface, and is empty when pressed (there is a pause in-between pulse beats at indefinite pulse counts). The following pulse beats also indicate *Rlung* disorder:
> Though long in continuum yet empty when pressed*
> Though short in continuum yet empty when pressed*
> Though soft yet empty when pressed*
> Though thin yet empty when pressed*
> Though strong yet empty when pressed*
> Though slow yet empty when pressed*

		Though high yet empty when pressed*
		Though low yet empty when pressed*
(2)	*mKhris.Pa* disorder:	The pulse beats fast and is prominent, thin and taut, like rolled horse tail and does not halt when pressed. The following pulse beats also indicate *mKhris.Pa* disorder:

Though thin yet taut when pressed*

Though strong yet taut when pressed*

Though slow yet taut when pressed*

Though high yet taut when pressed*

Though low yet taut when pressed*

(3) **Bad.Kan disorder:** The pulse is unclear and deeply sunken; weak and slow. The following pulse beats also indicate *Bad.Kan* disorder:

Though long in continuum yet weak*

Though short in continuum yet weak*

Though thick yet weak*

Though thin yet weak*

Though low yet weak*

Though high yet weak*

(4) **Rlung and fever combined disorder:**
Empty yet fast

(5) **Bad.Kan and mKhris.Pa combined disorder:**
Sunken yet taut

(6) **Bad.Kan and Rlung combined disorder:**
Empty and slow

(7) **Hot caused Bad.Kan sMug.Po:**
Thick and full yet unclear under the left middle finger

Cold caused Bad.Kan sMug.Po:
Thin and declining*

(8) **Blood disorder:** Protruding and rolling (refer to pregnancy pulse listed under seven wondrous pulse examination)

(9) **Lymph disorder:** Trembling and moves slower with difficulty

(10) **Microorganism:** Perceives like bound yet beats flatly

(11) **Skin diseases/leprosy:** Unclear, trembling and flick or low yet trembling and moves slower with difficulty*

(b) Seven contagious fever pulses

(1) **Disturbed fever:** Thick, overflowing, protruding, and rolling

(2) **Spread fever:** Thin, firm, and taut

(3)	Influenza:	Thin and fast
(4)	Infections:	Perceives like bound yet alternates from strong to weak or empty to thin and beats flat and dual
(5)	*gZer.Thung⁰*:	Short in continuum yet beats like something blowing inside the arteries
(6)	Compounded poison:	Coarse, fast, and fluctuates yet unclear and sunken
(7)	Meat poisoning:	Thin and fast yet occasionally unclear and sunken or is particularly unclear at the site of the affected organ's representation area at the radial artery

(c) Six temporal pulse beat

(1)	Unripened fever:	Thin, fast, and fluctuates like *Rlung*
(2)	High fever:	Strong and taut yet rolls when pressed
	Contagious fever:	Strong and coarse yet short in continuum*
	Throat and muscle inflammation:	
		Superficial yet taut at the deeper level and trembles internally*
(3)	Empty fever:	Empty when pressed yet beats fast
(4)	Hidden fever:	Low yet taut
	Cold prominent hidden fever:	Sunken and slow
(5)	Chronic fever:	The pulse beats thin and taut. In addition, the pulse may also beat in one of the following ways: Though long in continuum, pulse beats low* Though short in continuum, pulse beats low* Though thick pulse beats low* Though thin pulse beats low* Though fast pulse beats low*
	A very chronic fever:	Beats low yet long in continuum and taut*
(6)	Complicated fever:	Thin but beats fast at the deeper level
	Complicated lymph combined cold disorder:	Thin, empty, and fast*

(d) Seven hot disorders associated to the site

(1)	Septic wounds:	Thick, firm, and fast
(2)	**Infliction of wounds caused by weapons (foreign bodies, bullets, etc.):**	The pulse is unclear yet beats dual in accor-

dance with the side of the body that is injured

(3)	**Injury to head's muscle:**	Beats stronger underneath the index fingers
(4)	**Injury to head's bone:**	Beats taut underneath the middle fingers
(5)	**Injury to brain:**	Beats faster underneath the ring fingers[10]
(6)	**Internal pus formation:**	Trembles yet thin, fast, and, tender, rise of heat at the spot
(7)	**External pus formation:**	Same as above

(e) Six internal cold disorders

(1)	**Fresh indigestion:**	Thick and firm
(2)	**Chronic indigestion:**	Weak and thin
(3)	**Tumor:**	The pulse is weak and unclear in accordance with the organ that is affected or thin yet beats hard at the deeper level when pressed stronger to feel bone
	Rlung **tumor:**	Though empty pulse perceives like bound and hard*
	mKhris.Pa **tumor:**	Though thin pulse beats taut and hard*
	Blood tumor:	Though thick pulse beats strong and hard*
(4)	*sKya.rBab* **(initial stage edema):**	
		Thin, sunken, and tight at the deeper level
(5)	*'Or* **(second stage edema):**	Same as above
(6)	*dMu.Chu* **(last stage edema):**	Same as above
	Cold edema:	Low yet slow and trembles occasionally
	Rlung **edema:**	Thick, trembling, and empty when pressed*
	mKhris.Pa **edema:**	Thin, taut, and trembling*

(f) Two secondary cold disorders

(1)	**Vomiting:**	Weak underneath the index fingers
(2)	**Diarrhea:**	Weak underneath the ring fingers

(g) Two Secondary Hot Disorders

(1)	**Vomiting:**	Weak underneath the ring fingers
(2)	**Diarrhea:**	Weak underneath the index fingers

(h) Clearing the six misconceptions

The pulse of blood and *Rlung* disorders can be mistaken for one another due to a floating beat, yet if examined carefully:

(1)	Fresh blood disorder:	Though floating, taut and firm when pressed
(2)	*Rlung* disorder:	Though floating, does not feel when pressed and is empty

The pulse of high and empty fevers can be mistaken for one another due to a fast beat, yet if examined carefully:

(3)	High fever:	Strong and taut when pressed
(4)	Empty fever:	Empties when pressed

The pulse of *Bad.Kan* and chronic blood disorders can be mistaken for one another due to being sunken deeply, yet if examined carefully:

(5)	*Bad.Kan* disorder:	Declining and slow
(6)	Chronic blood disorder:	Beats stronger

Note: The pulse beats marked with an asterisk above are added here from other books to give readers more information.

(i) Ten additional pulse beats

The following pulse beats are also added here from other books (except the four critical points):

(1) **Blood dominant high blood pressure:**
Overflowing, thick, and strong
(2) ***Rlung* dominant high blood pressure:**
In addition, empties when pressed
(3) **Chronic high blood pressure:** Sunken yet strong and taut
(4) **Fresh fever:** Though thick, beats high and fast
Though thin, high and fast
Though strong, high and fast
Though taut, high and fast
Though short in continuum, high and fast; all indicate fresh fever.
(5) **Dysentery:** Fast, taut, and weak underneath the ring fingers
(6) **Involuntary discharge of semen:**
Unclear underneath both the ring fingers or sunken and slow
(7) **Vaginal discharge:** Same as above
(8) **Impaired digestive heat:** Halts beat underneath the middle fingers

(9) Diseases of vital and vessel organs:
Halts beat at the site of the respective organ's representation area at the radial artery

(10) *Rlung* disorder: May halt beat underneath all the fingers

(j) Four Critical Points for Determining the Hot and Cold Disorders:

- Whether the rate of the pulse is more or less than those previously mentioned (healthy and unhealthy pulse rates), firm and taut indicates a fever.
- Though the rate of the pulse is more than those previously mentioned (healthy and unhealthy pulse rates), empty and loose indicates a cold disorder.
- Though the rate of the pulse, which is more than those previously mentioned (healthy and unhealthy pulse rates) is an indication of a hot disorder, in reality, it should be understood as a cold disorder if it empties when pressed stronger.
- Though the rate of the pulse, which is less than those previously mentioned (healthy and unhealthy pulse rates), is an indication of a cold disorder, in reality, it should be understood as a hot disorder if there is firmness when pressed stronger.

Death Pulse

Certain pulse characteristics are associated with the terminal cases. These characteristics ensue due to the degeneration of the vital life force, elements, and energies, as well as the loss of bodily functions. Under this topic, the change in characteristics of pulse, missing pulse, interpretation of missing pulse for a healthy person, pause in pulse, and recovery pulse are explained in order.

Change in characteristics of pulse:

Rlung disorder:
Empty and thick, yet trembles and halts at uncertain time like a flapping flag

mKhris.Pa disorder:
Very fast and trembling like a soaring hawk's vibrating tip of the tail

Bad.Kan disorder:
Slow and trembling like uneven dripping of water

Rlung and *mKhris.Pa* combined disorder:
Strong yet deeply sunken and halts like a fish suddenly darting up to eat food[11]

Bad.Kan and *mKhris.Pa* combined disorder:

Overflowing, long in continuum, and halts like the jumping of a frog

Bad.Kan and Rlung combined disorder:

The number of beats and halting varies like a common sparrow picking its food from the ground and then taking rest

Tri-Nyes.Pa disorder:

Empty, slow, fluctuating, and trembling like saliva flowing steadily from an old bull's mouth.

- The pulse beats weak and unclear or very thin for a strongly built person who is struck suddenly by an acute throat or muscle inflammation or abdominal cramps, or other ailments
- An appearance of overflowing and strong pulse beat for a very chronic and emaciated patient
- An appearance of strong and overflowing, hot disorder's pulse for a patient suffering from a cold disorder
- An appearance of weak and sunken, cold disorder's pulse for a patient suffering from a hot disorder
- An appearance of a healthy pulse for a patient with acute lung infection
- An appearance of a healthy pulse for a patient with acute meat poisoning
- An appearance of a healthy pulse for a patient with acute abdominal cramps of solidifying Bad.Kan (mucus)
- An appearance of a healthy pulse for a patient with acute abdominal cramps of solidifying bile

Missing pulse:

Missing pulses should be examined in correlation with the vital organs, vessel organs, and the five sense organs. The following signs indicate impending death:

- An absence of the heart and small intestine pulse correlated with a black tongue and staring indicate the person will die in one day.
- An absence of the lungs and large intestine pulse correlated with sunken nostrils and the turning upward of hair in the nostrils indicate the person will die in two days.
- An absence of the liver and gall bladder pulse correlated with the eyeballs turning upward and rising up or circling of the eyebrows in different directions indicate the person will die in three days.
- An absence of the spleen and stomach pulse correlated with the fall of lower lip and the sinking of the xiphoid appendix indicate the person will die in five days.
- An absence of the right and left kidney, urinary bladder and reproduc-

tive organ's pulse correlated with the loss of whirring sound, and back of earlobes sticking to the head indicate the person will die in eight days.

Interpretation of missing pulse for healthy person: [12]

- An absence of the heart pulse indicates the person will die in one month.
- An absence of the lung pulse indicates the person will die in two months.
- An absence of the liver pulse indicates the person will die in three months.
- An absence of the spleen pulse indicates the person will die in five months.
- An absence of the kidney pulse indicates the person will die in eight months.

Pause in pulse:

If there is a regular halt of the pulse beat on the same count one hundred times, death is to be expected. Halting of the pulse beat before and after five counts is an indication of proximate and distal death, respectively.

Near death:	Thick yet halts on same count
Distant death:	Thin yet halts on same count
Near death:	Halts on odd number
Distant death:	Halts on even number
Near death:	Halts the pulse of vital organ
Distant death:	Halts the pulse of vessel organ

Recovery pulse:

The change of pulse from thick to thin following pulses indicates a patient is recovering from his or her illness. It is also said that the more the pulse is thick and soft, the greater the chance of the patient's survival.

- Thin becomes thick
- Short in continuum becomes long in continuum
- Sunken (low) becomes superficial (high)
- Taut becomes loose
- Empty becomes taut
- Firm becomes soft
- High becomes low
- Disappearance of the halting of pulse beat

- Disappearance of missing pulse

Evil Spirits Pulse

The pulse beats irregularly with multiple changes at the right and left radial artery or upper (vital organs) and lower (vessel organs) sites or pulsates from a hot to cold disorder and vice versa plus halts, pulls or beats dual in an uncertain count with sudden and frequent change.

These indicate the harmful influence of evil spirits on the patient. To ward of these influences, a patient is advised to perform religious practices like circumambulating holy sites, making prostration, reading religious scriptures, saving the lives of animals, giving donations to schools and hospitals, and helping the poor and needy, etc., to build up virtuous actions. Medicines will be ineffective if they are given prior to the patient's performance of these religious practices.

Vital Life Force (Bla) Pulse

To determine a patient's life span, the life force pulse is read on the ulnar artery. The basis on which our life depends is *Bla*.

If the pulse beat of the *Bla* is stable, there is no impending harm for a life, whereas unstable *Bla* indicates the uncertainty of life itself. If the *Bla* pulse is missing, the person will not be expected to survive; however, by receiving long life initiation, performing pujas, reciting life-prolonging mantras, and summoning back the *Bla* by performing special rituals, the patient can be saved from death. This is indicated by the return of the life force pulse beat.

The number of beats that the life force pulses remains consistent (i.e., without any change or variation) equals the number of years in that person's life span.[13] Refer to Figure 2.1.2 and the explanation given under *Site of Pulse Examination* for more information.

Summary

The following things are detected more clearly by pulse examination:

- The diseases pertaining to the five vital organs
- Whether the patient will live or not

A critical point about pulse examination follows in Tibetan and English.[14] The verse in Tibetan is:

rTsa.Ni Gar.mKhan Gyi Lag.Pa 'Dra
Kha.sMra Thogs.Pa gCig.Kyang Med
rTsa gTing.Shed Che.Ba Tsha.Ba Yin

gTing.Shed Med.Na Grang.Ba Yin

The English translation is:

The pulse is like a hand (a gesture that changes with each movement) of a dancer

There is nothing from which (a physician) can detect

Conclude a hot disorder, if the pulse beats stronger at the deeper level

Whereas a cold disorder from a pulse that is weak at the deeper lever.

To gain confidence in pulse examination, a physician needs a lot of practice and requires full concentration. Also, the freshness and wellbeing of both the physical and mental health is necessary to have clear judgment. Experience is most important of all. Therefore, the more one sees patients, the more one gains experience, and for that, one really needs to pay attention to the different beats of the pulse.

CHAPTER TWO

DIAGNOSIS BY URINE EXAMINATION

Urine is like a mirror that reflects the features of disorders. Since it is an end product of the body fluids, it carries information about any disorders. The physician visually examines the reflection of color, steam, odor, and bubbles, and many other characteristics from the patient's first morning mid-stream urine. In general, visual examination consists of examining the following subjects:

- Complexion of the skin
- Color and texture of the blood (in sputum, vomiting, urine, and stool)
- Nails
- Sputum
- Feces
- Physical structure
- Abnormalities on the body and other general conditions

The examination of the urine is explained under the following eight sections.

Prerequisite Conditions

It is important for both the patient and the physician to observe certain preliminaries prior to the day of the actual urine examination. For instance, the night before the examination, the patient should refrain from the following things to avoid altering the urine's characteristics:

Excessive tea, coffee, and pork: to avoid false characteristics of *Rlung* disorder

Meat and alcohol:* to avoid false characteristics of *mKhris.Pa* disorder

Excessive sweets, unripened fruits, stale and greasy foods, and buttermilk:*
to avoid false characteristics of *Bad.Kan* disorder

Strong physical exertions like jogging:*

to avoid false characteristics of blood and *Rlung* disturbances

Insufficient sleep:*

to avoid false characteristics of *Rlung* disorder

Fasting or lack of food:[1]*   (Same as above)

Exhaustion from sexual indulgence:*   (Same as above)

Mental/emotional stress:*   (Same as above)

Vitamins: to avoid altering the urine's color

***Note:** The physician should also refrain from those conditions marked with an asterisk so that he or she can more accurately diagnose the patient.

The patient should collect the first morning mid-stream urine. Urine should not be used which has an influence of foods and beverages that is taken at night (the first urine after the consumption of a meal). For example, meat and alcohol taken between seven to eight P.M. may take about four hours to digest according to one's metabolism. The post-digestion essences absorbed from the food and beverage will naturally influence the urine. Therefore, he or she must eliminate that urine by midnight. Unless the patient has eliminated the urine that has an influence of meat and beverage, he or she may be misdiagnosed with a "hot" disorder. Patients who are coming to see physician must be advised properly regarding this matter.

Time of Urine Examination

The time for examining urine is in the morning when the sun's rays strike the container of the urine. Daylight examination is also right for clear observation of the intensity of color, steam, and many other characteristics of the urine. It must not be examined under electric light as its color may not be clearly observed.

Container for the Urine

For examination, the urine is poured into a cup that is white on the inside to prevent discoloration of the urine. The container must be clean and devoid of any contamination and should not be of clay, copper, iron, or anything that will affect the color of the urine. The urine is stirred with sticks to facilitate observation of changes. Urine can also be examined in transparent glass containers and bottles. Figure 2.2.1 shows a typical container of urine and two stirring sticks.

Origination of Sediments

Urine, as one of the three waste products, is eliminated from time to time. The foods and beverages one takes are decomposed, digested, and separated into thick and thin waste products in the intestines by the three digestive heats. The thick products become feces and the thin products become urine. The absorbed post-digestive nutritional essences become blood in the liver. The waste from the blood is then stored in the gall bladder as bile. The refined portion of bile becomes lymph and the waste becomes sediment. Hence, the sediment in urine originates from the blood and *mKhris.Pa* sites, the liver and gall bladder, which are the two organs that induce heat in the body. The higher the body temperature, the more sediment will appear in the urine. When the body temperature decreases, so do the sediments. Thus, the intensity of the sediment deposits in the urine depends on body temperature.

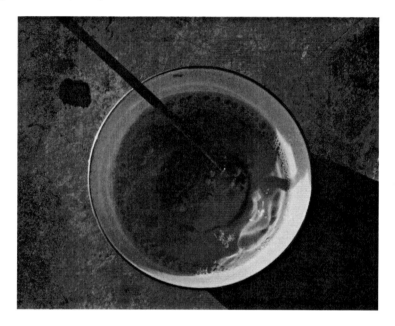

Figure 2.2.1: A Close up View of the Container and Stirring Stick

Healthy Urine

Under this topic, the characteristics of balanced and healthy urine and urine characteristics according to age difference are explained.

The Characteristics of Balanced and Healthy Urine:

- Clear light-yellow color
- Steam of moderate intensity and duration
- Medium-sized bubbles when stirred vigorously
- Moderate and properly diffused sediments

- Spring water-like moderate scum
- Disappearance of bubbles beginning concentrically from the periphery to the center while the steam begins to evaporate
- Change of color to whitish-yellow after stirring

Urine Characteristics According to Age Difference:

Infant (breast milk dependent):	Post-change (after stirring or when urine is cold) whitish and turbid
Child:	Whitish due to *Bad.Kan* as a natural condition of childhood
Adult:	Yellowish due to *mKhris.Pa* as a natural condition of adulthood
Aged:	Slightly bluish due to *Rlung* as a natural condition of old age
Pregnant:	Bluish in color and containing sediment

Unhealthy Urine

If the characteristics of the urine are opposite to that of the healthy urine, it is considered unhealthy. These characteristics are explained under the general and specific examinations. The determination of any disorder is made by careful analysis of many factors including visual examination of the body, pulse examination, and the details listed below regarding general and specific examinations of the urine.

General Examination

The urine should be examined at three different temperatures: warm, lukewarm, and cold. The physician observes the just-voided urine for its color, steam, odor, and bubbles. The sediments and scum are observed when the urine is lukewarm. Finally, when the urine is cooled, the time of changes, modes of change, and the post-change characteristics are noted. The characteristics of the urine and their associated disorders follow.

When Urine Is Warm

(a) Color:

Rlung disorder:	Bluish (and thin) like spring water
mKhris.Pa disorder:	Yellow
Bad.Kan disorder:	White and turbid like milk (indigestion, etc.)
Blood disorder:	Red-like blood (proliferation of blood in liver, etc.)
Lymph disorder:	Whitish-pink

Bad.Kan sMug.Po:	Brown and fetid
Lymph and *Rlung* combined disorder:	
	Brownish-blue
Bad.Kan and *mKhris.Pa* conflicting disorder[2]:	
	Brownish-yellow
Black lymph disorder[3]:	Brownish-black
Highly toxic infections:	Same as above
Bad.Kan and *Rlung* combined disorder:	
	Bluish-pale
Rlung and *mKhris.Pa* combined disorder:	
	Bluish-yellow
Rlung and blood combined disorder:	
	Bluish-red
mKhris.Pa and *Bad.Kan* combined disorder:	
	Yellowish-pale
Blood and *mKhris.Pa* combined disorder:	
	Reddish-yellow
Bad.Kan and blood combined disorder:	
	Whitish-red
Acute infections:	Thick, turbid, and yellowish-black like mustard oil
Highly increased *mKhris.Pa* disorders, including hepatitis:	
	Same as above
Spread fever (if red color is stronger):	
	Reddish-yellow, thick and fetid
Disturbed fever (if yellow color is stronger):	
	Reddish-yellow, thick and fetid
Poisoning:	Like ink (black) or like a rainbow

(b) Steam:

High fever:	Plentiful and intense (like a steam of a hot spring, that obscures the urine's color)
Hidden fever:	Light yet remains for a long time
Chronic fever:	Same as above
Bad.Kan disorder:	Light and fast disappearing
Rlung disorder:	Same as above
Cold disorder:	Same as above
Hot and cold combined disorder:	Alternates from much to low or vise-versa

(c) Odor:

High fever:	Foul
Cold disorder:	Light or no odor
Indigestion:	Smells of the food which has not digested

mKhris.Pa disorder:	Burnt odor
Blood disorder:	Smells of blood
Pus:	Smells of pus
dMu.Chu:	Smells of radish leaves*
Rlung disorder:	Smells of oxide*
Bad.Kan disorder:	Smells of lice*
Tri-*Nyes.Pa* disorder:	Smells of Adipose tissue*
Muscle inflammation:	Smells of brain*

Note: I did not see any explanation so far about the factors marked with an asterisk above. However, I present them here with the belief that I may find their underlying secrets in the near future.

(d) Bubbles

Rlung disorder:	Bluish and protruding; bubbles look large, like the eyes of *mZo.Mo* (This is explained in Part One, Chapter Five, Note 5)
Chest congestion:	Bluish and tiny
Spleen *Rlung* disorder:	Bubbles appear whitish, large and rolled
mKhris.Pa disorder:	Thin and tiny like the eyes of a fish with many bubbles that are tinted yellow and which disappear quickly
Inflammation:	Same as above with the addition of crackling sounds when the bubbles disappear
Bad.Kan disorder:	Whitish, frothy, and sticky, like saliva thrown in water which remains static on the surface of the urine
Blood disorder:	Bubbles have a reddish tint
Poisoning:	Variously colored like a rainbow
Hot or cold spread disorder[4]:	Spreads immediately from the center to the edges of container like a flock of pigeons who go off in all directions due to being dive-bombed by a hawk

When Urine is Lukewarm

(a) Sediments:

Rlung disorder:	Like goat's hair thrown in water, can be taken off the urine with the tip of the spoon yet in reality there is none

Blood and *mKhris.Pa* combined disorder:

Like cotton thrown in water which swings mostly in the center and obscures the bottom of the container

Bad.Kan disorder:	Like residue of wheat flour strained in a strainer[5]
Cold disorder:	Same as above
Pneumonia, lung infections, etc,:	Cloud-like (whitish-blue with black tint underneath and elongated edge) swinging
Pus:	Pus-like
Kidneys disorder:	Sand-like whitish-blue particles that settle at the bottom of the container
Heart and lung, upper body disorder:	
	Appears on the surface
Liver and spleen, middle body disorder:	
	Appears in the middle
Kidneys and intestines, lower body disorder:	
	Settles at the bottom
***Rlung* agitated hot and cold bodily constituents disorder:**	
	Dried yogurt-like white particles that thinly cover the surface
Hot disorder:	Thick
Cold disorder:	Light
Lung and heart disorder:	Reddish with red tinted sediments on the surface
Influenza:	Same as above

(b) Scum:

Hot disorder:	Thick
Cold disorder:	Light
Tumor:	Separates into many pieces when still and not stirred

Note: Though a thick layer of scum is an indication of a hot disorder, if it can be taken off the surface with the tip of the spoon, it is called wild grease and the intensity of the hot disorder may not be strong. When burnt, if it smells of a burnt *rTsam.Pa* (Tibetan food of roasted barley flour), it is just an indication of not digesting butter or greasy foods, etc. It will cease by itself, and thus there is no need for treatment. However, if it does not smell like burnt *rTsam.Pa*, it indicates dissolving bodily constituents by fever and must be treated.

When Urine Is Cold

(a) Time of Changes:

Hot disorder:	Urine characteristics change from clear to turbid before vapor disappears and the urine cools

Cold disorder:	Urine characteristics change from turbid to clear after the disappearance of vapor and the urine cools
Hot and cold in balanced or healthy urine:	
	Both the change in urine characteristics and the disappearance of vapor come at the same time
During winter:	Changes come immediately
During spring and autumn:	Changes come slower (it is slower than winter and faster than summer because of variations in the temperature during these seasons.)
During summer:	Changes come slowly

(b) Modes of Change:

Fresh fever:	Changes in urine come from the bottom center to the top like boiling water
Chronic fever:	Changes in urine come from the edges of the container to the center, like when a string is pulled
Cold disorder:	Changes in urine come gradually from the edges of the container
Hot and cold conflicting disorder:	Sediments disappear before the urine changes
Spread fever[6]:	Changes do not come
Chronic cold disorder:	Same as above
Chronic cold diarrhea:	Same as above
Evil spirit caused disorder:	Same as above
Excessive sexual indulgence:	Same as above
Black **lymph disorder:**	Same as above

(c) Post-Change Characteristics:

Hot disorder:	More turbid
Cold disorder:	Clear
Kidney disorder:	Numerous and rotten-like sediments

Specific Examination

During a specific examination, the characteristics of hot, cold, *Rlung, mKhris.Pa*, and *Bad.Kan* disorders, and clearing the misconceptions are explained. There are five types of misconceptions that must be explained: color, modes of changes, bubbles, scum, and the type of diseases.

(a) The characteristics of a hot disorder:

Color:	Red or yellow and thick
Steam:	Plentiful, intense, and long lasting
Odor:	Fetid
Bubbles:	Thin and tiny like the eyes of a fish with many bubbles, a yellowish tint, and quickly disappearing
Scum:	Thick
Sediments:	Thick and swings in the middle
Time of changes:	Changes from clear to turbid before the disappearance of vapor and while the urine is warm
Post-change characteristics:	Thick and brownish or cinnabar-like redness in the bottom of the urine

(b) The characteristics of cold disorder:

Color:	White or bluish and thin
Steam:	Light
Odor:	Light
Bubbles:	Large or plentiful bubbles that disappear slowly
Scum:	Light
Sediments:	Light and thin
Time of changes:	Changes from turbid to clear after the disappearance of vapor
Post-change characteristics:	Bluish and thin

(c) The characteristics of *Rlung* disorder:
- Bluish and thin like spring water
- Large bubbles when stirred

(d) The characteristics of *mKhris.Pa* disorder:
- Yellowish-red with lots of steam
- Fetid with quickly disappearing tiny bubbles

(e) The characteristics of *Bad.Kan* disorder:
- Whitish with light odor and vapor
- Saliva-like bubbles

(f) Clearing the misconceptions about color:

Whitish-blue with thick sediments: Though this looks like a cold disorder because of the color, in reality, it is a deep-seated hot disorder due to the additional sediments

Reddish-yellow with light odor and no sediments:

Though this looks like a hot disorder because of the color, in reality, it is a cold disorder

(g) Clearing the misconceptions about the modes of change:

Urine with hot characteristics and slow changes:

Reddish-yellow in color and other hot characteristics such as steam, odor, etc., are present, yet the changes come slowly and after the disappearance of warmth and vapor. This indicates a hidden fever.

Urine with cold characteristics and quick changes:

Whitish-blue in color and other cold characteristics are present, yet the changes come quickly and before the disappearance of warmth and vapor. This also indicates a hidden fever.

(h) Clearing the misconceptions about bubbles:

Hot characteristic urine with no bubbles:

Reddish-yellow in color and most of the hot characteristics are present, yet the absent of bubbles after stirring is an indication of a deeply buried internal hot disorder.

Cold characteristic urine with no bubbles:

Whitish-blue in color, and most of the cold characteristics are present, yet the absent of bubbles after stirring is an indication of a chronic cold disorder or chronic cold diarrhea.

(i) Clearing the misconceptions about scum:

Hot characteristic urine with thick scum:

Reddish-yellow in color, and other hot characteristics are present. In addition, a thick layer of oily scum indicates dissolving bodily constituents by fever.

Cold characteristic urine with thick scum:

Whitish-blue in color and other cold characteristics are present. In addition, a thick layer of oily scum indicates the improper digestion of butter by cold disorder.

- A thick layer of scum-like milk cream is also an indication of not digesting butter.
- A thick layer of scum-like honey is an indication of not digesting butter and milk.
- A thick layer of yellowish-black scum is an indication of not digesting meat.
- A thick layer of scum-like egg yolk is an indication of not digesting fats and nutritious foods.

(j) Clearing the misconceptions about the type of diseases:

The urine of an empty fever and the rise of blood temperature including blood infections can be mistaken for one another due to the red color, yet if examined carefully:

Empty fever: The remnant of fever increased by *Rlung's* urine is red, yet it is clear, and thin with slightly larger bubbles.

High blood temperature: Though red, it is turbid and thick with many sediments and vapor, with smaller bubbles.

The urine of *Bad.Kan sMug.Po* and black lymph disorder can be mistaken for one another due to brownish color, yet if examined carefully:

Bad.Kan sMug.Po: Though brown in color, it is thick and fetid.

Black lymph disorder: Though brown in color, it is clear with a whitish-pink tint in the edges and has a light odor.

The urine of kidneys, liver, and spleen ailments can be mistaken for one another due to the red color, yet if examined carefully:

Kidney ailment: Though red, it is turbid and the sediments settle in the bottom.

Liver ailment: Though red, it has a reddish-black or reddish-pale tint with sediments dispersed throughout the urine.

Spleen ailment: Though red, it has a greenish tint or is clear with sediments in the middle.

The urine of a hidden fever, *Bad.Kan* and *Rlung* combined disorder, and cold disorder can be mistaken for one another due to a bluish color, yet if examined carefully:

Hidden fever: Though bluish, it contains thin and fast disappearing bubbles with thick sediments.

Bad.Kan and Rlung combined disorder:

         Though bluish in color, it contains large and stable or slowly disappearing bubbles with few or no sediments.

Cold disorder: Bluish-pale with thin sediments.

Death Urine

Like the pulse, urine also reflects certain characteristics associated with terminal cases. These characteristics in urine come due to degeneration of vital life force, elements, energies, stamina, and bodily functions. This will be explained below in accordance with the hot and cold disorders and the type of diseases.

Hot Disorder:
Color: Like blood
Odor: Smells like rotten leather
Sediments: Thick

Despite resorting to the four waters, [7] there is no improvement in the patient's condition nor change in urine characteristics except sediment. Both of these indicate a terminal hot disorder.

Cold Disorder:
Color: Bluish
         With no steam, smell, sediments, bubbles, or taste

Despite resorting to the four fires, [8] (both) no improvement in the patient's condition nor change in urine characteristics.

Rlung Disorder:
Color: Boiled vegetable-like bluish-black
         Separation of fluids and sediments

mKhris.Pa Disorder:
Color: Concentrated decoction of rheum species, yellow and putrid

Separation of fluids and sediments

Blood Disorder:
Color: Cinnabar-like red and putrid
                                Separation of fluids and sediments

Bad.Kan Disorder:
Color: Spoiled milk, whitish-blue
                                Separation of fluids and sediments

Poisoning:
Color: Ink-like black
                                Separation of fluids and sediments

Tri-Nyes.Pa Disorder: Passing of urine, putrid with no illness to the
                                kidneys is called putrefaction of internal
                                humors.

Evil Spirits Urine

The notion of harmful influences from evil spirits as well as the possession of human beings by the evil spirits is well accepted in many Asian countries, including Tibet. An oracle would be a good example to support the notion of evil spirits urine. For more information, read *Tibetan Buddhist Medicine & Psychiatry, the Diamond Healing* by Terry Clifford.

To assess the harmful influences of evil spirits in urine, the physician views the urine as a mirror that reflects their influences in the form of a shadow. For male patients, the container of urine is viewed as a turtle lying on its back, with its right side to the East, left to West, head to South, and tail to North. For female patients, the container of the urine is viewed as a turtle lying face downward with its left side to the East, right to West, head to South, and tail to North. The side of the container/cup onto which the man and woman urinates is also viewed as East and West, respectively.

Thereafter, to examine the shadow of the evil spirits from the four directions and the four cardinal directions, a grid with nine partitions (Tib: *Ling.Tshe dGu*; Eng: A lattice with nine squares or rectangles) is made, putting the four thin sticks on the urine container. The elements Wood (East), Fire (South), Metal (West), Water (North), and Earth (the four cardinal directions) govern the directions. The manifestation of the different evil spirits and their remedies is ascertained from the following characteristics in a particular grid with the aid of the "Turtle Graphs." Refer to Figures 2.2.2 and 2.2.3 below which show the grids for a male (turtle lying on its back) and female (turtle lying face downward). The characteristics of evil spirit urine follow with (*Ling.Tshe dGu*) a lattice with nine squares or rectangles.

The Characteristics of Evil Spirit Urine:

- Fast disappearance of bubbles from a particular grid location before the bubbles disappear in another location
- Slow disappearance of bubbles from a particular grid after the others
- Non-disappearance of bubbles
- Appearance of fish-eye-like bubbles in a particular grid
- Appearance of a suture-like line from bubbles[9] in a particular grid when the urine is still and not stirred
- Appearance of a reflection like a peacock's feather, raised flag, iron chain, the tip of spears, and many others from bubbles, sediments, or scum in a particular grid reflect a particular spirit.

A Lattice with Nine Squares or Rectangles (Ling.Tshe dGu):

Gods: The appearance of any of the above characteristics in the "Gods" location is attributed to the influence of paternal ancestors or the presence of one's worshipping protector. To pacify this influence, the patient should perform copious religious rites to please the protector.

Humans: The appearance of any of the above characteristics is attributed to the influence of male and female demons. To pacify their influence, the patient must offer articles to please them as well as accumulate merit by performing religious ceremonies (rites).

Spirits: The influence of universally known spirits, like kings' spirits, are pacified by ritually offering cakes (gTor.Ma) and performing the crossed thread ritual (mDos) of five colors: red, green, blue, white, and yellow. See Figure 2.2.4 below.

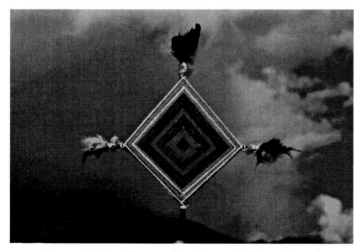

Figure 2.2.4: mDos used in Crossed Thread Ritual

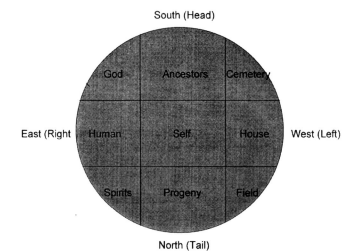

Figure 2.2.2. Mirror of the Male Urine: Turtle Lying on Its Back.

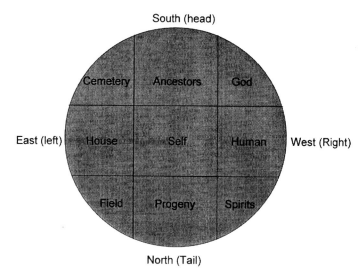

Figure 2.2.3 Mirror of the Female Urine: Turtle Lying Face Downward

Ancestors: To eliminate the influence of paternal and maternal ancestors born as ghost spirits due to attachment to property (e.g. houses, fields, wealth) and of ghost-compelled sorcerers, perform the crossed thread ritual (*mDos*), worshipping the tutelary deities of the family and offering small round pills made from *rTsam.Pa* (roasted barley flour) for karmic retribution.

Self: Appearance of any of the above characteristics indicate harm from a spirit accompanying a person with whom the patient is emotionally close.[10] The influence

94

of this spirit is pacified by diverting its direction and performing wrathful religious practices.

Progeny: To pacify the influence of the spirits of maternal relative side, the patient must offer cakes, effigies, and crossed thread rituals to them.

Cemetery: To pacify the arisal of misfortunes from spirits abiding in a cemetery and from an improper funeral ceremony, the patient must ritually change the site of the burning place, river burial place, or graveyard.

Home: Harm from *Naga,* [11] *gNyan,* [12] or *Sa.bDag*[13] is pacified by ritually burying a sacred pot containing consecrated objects and various sorts of medicines on the particular ground inhabited by the spirits and by liberating them in a peaceful way.

Field: The influence of *Naga, gNyan,* and *Sa.bDag* are pacified in the ways mentioned above.

Summary

The following things are detected more clearly by urine examination:

- The diseases pertaining to six vessel organs
- The differences between the hot and cold disorders

A critical point about urine examination follows in Tibetan and English. [14] The verse in Tibetan is:

Chu.Ni 'Ja'. Tshon Gyi Ri.Mo 'Dra
Mig.Gis mThong.Yang brTag.Thabs dKa'
Ku.Ya mThug.Na Tsha.Ba Yin
Ku.Ya Srab.Na Grang.Ba Yin.

The English translation is:

The reflections in urine are like a rainbow
Though a (physician) sees it is difficult to diagnose
Conclude a hot disorder if the sediments are plentiful,
And a cold disorder if the sediments are thin.

When I was working under Dr. Yeshi Dhonden in 1980s, I paid great attention to his practice with great curiosity in becoming a physician like him. Unlike some Tibetan physicians, he pays great emphasis to the examination of both the patients' pulse and urine. I used to wonder about and admire his never tiring energy in seeing patients, as well as the confidence and the skills he gained in the practice. He has traveled many time to Europe and visits the United States every year to conduct research with Western physicians, as well as for conferences, seminars, and consultations. I have now realized why he was paying similar emphasis for the pulse and urine examinations from the summaries given at the end of both the diagnosis by pulse and urine examinations and the critical points mentioned by Yuthog Yonten Gonpo. See Figure 2.2.5 below for Dr. Yeshi Dhonden.

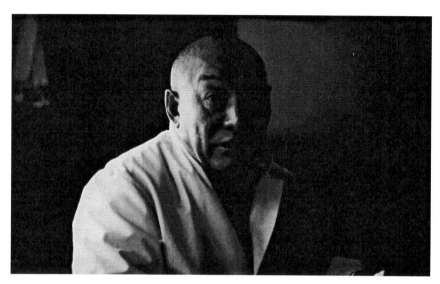

Figure 2.2.5: Dr. Yeshe Dhonden, the former personal physician to His Holiness the XIVth Dalai Lama and an author of *Health through Balance and Healing from the Source*.

To gain confidence in urine examination, it is necessary to have a lot of practice and it requires full concentration. Therefore, the more one examines patients' urine, the more experiences one gains. It is also essential for the physician to pay attention to all the features reflected in the urine. In addition, the freshness of the senses and the wellbeing of both the physician's physical and mental health is necessary to have clear judgment.

CHAPTER THREE

SECONDARY DIAGNOSIS

The secondary diagnosis is part of the visual observation and is comprised of examining the person's nature, eyes, and the technique of examining the child's ear—twelve different subjects.

1. Examining the Person's Nature

The nature of the person can be *Rlung*, *mKhris.Pa*, *Bad.Kan*, or dual combinations of *Rlung* and *mKhris.Pa*, *Bad.Kan* and *Rlung*, *Bad.Kan* and *mKhris.Pa*, or of all three *Nyes.Pa*. The primary constituents of an offspring depend on its father's sperm and mother's ovum. The lifestyle and eating and drinking habits of the mother while pregnant also play a great role in determining her offspring's nature. This also implies that the person is susceptible to disorders related to the nature to which one belongs.

Person of *Rlung* Nature:

- Lacks brightness in hair and body with dark complexion
- Unable to endure cold and wind and desires warm environment
- Fluctuating and unstable memory, intelligence, behavior, love for one's friend, is fidgety
- Lacks wealth, *Bad.Kan* constituents, and is a light sleeper
- Thin, stooped, small in stature, and short life
- Joints give crackling sound when one moves
- Likes talking, dancing, singing, laughing, hunting, challenges, and fighting
- Likes sweet, sour, bitter, and hot tastes[1]
- Mentally elated and is rough
- Like a vulture[2], craves for meat
- Like a fox, is elated and conceits wrong
- Like a hawk, likes to kill and watch for its prey

97

Person of *mKhris.Pa* Nature:

- Great thirst and hunger
- Great digestive and body heat, little tolerance to heat
- Desires cool environment
- Yellowish hair and body
- Much sweating and malodorous
- Mentally sharp, brave, and full of pride
- Likes using scent and ornament
- Likes sweet, bitter, astringent, and cooling powered foods and beverages
- Medium life, wealth and stature
- Like tiger, has great hunger
- Like monkey, craves food
- Like *yaksha* (harmful spirit), mentally sharp and has great pride

Person of *Bad.Kan* Nature:

- Has low digestive heat, cool bodies, and pale complexion
- Fat, stout, and erect posture
- Joints are not prominent
- Can endure hunger, thirst, heat, and mental torments
- Long life, much wealth, and thick sleeper
- Kind and hard to arouse anger from the depth of mire
- Likes hot, sour, astringent, and coarse powered foods and beverages
- Mentally firm, courageous, and speaks pleasant words
- Has smooth skin, generous, and honest
- Like a lion, joints are not prominent and has fair complexion
- Like the chief of elephants, who guides the herd, is corpulent and lives long

Classification of dual or all three *Nyes.Pa* combined natures are done from the blend of qualities mentioned above of *Rlung*, *mKhris.Pa*, and *Bad.Kan*. Among the seven natures, each subsequent order is considered superior to the preceding one.

2. Examining the Eyes

The eyes are in the nature of the fire element because of its connection to the liver and sight *mKhris.Pa*. The eyes are also considered flower of the liver. Therefore, whether one has a blood or *mKhris.Pa* disorder in the liver, it can be inferred from the eyes becoming red or yellow, respectively. The eyes see things because of sight *mKhris.Pa*, which is located in the eyes. The transmission of information between the eyes and brain take in the form of nerve impulses. It is also a function of one of the five-branch *Rlungs* called *Klu* (Kalachakra Tantra:

Moving *Rlung*). They are the branches of life-sustaining *Rlung*, which is located in the head. The function of life-sustaining *Rlung* is explained in Part One, Chapter Three, and under the topic Branch 1: Fifteen Afflictions.

To produce a visual sense consciousness, however three conditions are required. They are: (i) an empowering condition which is the eye sense faculty; (ii) an observed-object-condition which is a visible form, shape, or color; and (iii) an immediately preceding condition, a former moment of consciousness. The functions of the three conditions follow with the characteristics of eye disorders.

The Functions of Three Conditions

Eye sense faculty:	Apprehends visible form
Observed-object-condition:	Generates the object in the form of color or shape
Immediately preceding condition:	Knowing and luminosity

The Characteristics of Eye Disorders

***Rlung* disorder:**	Redness in sclera, swollen or tears
***mKhris.Pa* disorder:**	Yellow sclera
***Bad.Kan* disorder:**	Pale and weak eyesight
Acute *Rlung* disorder or brain damage:	Fixed gaze
Fever or blood disorder:	Redness in sclera
Anemia:	Pale inside the eyelids
Rise of bad blood: [3]	Very red
Poisoning or brain damage:	Pupil becomes bigger in size
Initial stage edema or kidneys disorder:	Swollen and puffy
Prolapsed liver disease of infant: [4]	Looks up
Measles:	Reddest at outer edge and sore

3. The Technique of Examining a Child's Ear

The ears are considered flowers of the kidneys, and the size of the ears and kidneys are said to be the same. When one is stricken with the kidneys' *Rlung* disorder, the symptoms associated are pain in the kidneys and waist region and loss of hearing. The ears hear sound because of nerve impulses. The nerve impulses are the function of the branch *Rlung* called Rus.sBal (Kalachakra Tantra: thoroughly moving *Rlung*). Like eyes, to produce a hearing sense consciousness, three conditions are required. The application is the same as the previously mentioned in the eyes' examination.

The pulses of earlobes are examined from the backside as a substitute for the radial artery for babies of twelve days to children of eight years old. Overall energies, including the movement of *Rlung* and blood, are just developing the pulses at the radial artery and do not provide clear information. The time of examining a child's ear follows with the methods of examining a child's ear.

The Time of Examining a Child's Ear:

The time for examination, the text says, is in the morning when the sun rises from the east. However, it is also right to examine during the day. Clean the ears before examining with wet towel. Then keep the patient faced to the sun to see clearly the different pulses of earlobes from the backside.

The Methods of Examining a Child's Ear:

The methods of examining organs and parts of the body at the backside of the left and right earlobes are the same as a pulse examination at the radial artery. Like a pulse examination, the site of the heart/small intestine and lungs/large intestine are reversed from left to right between the boys and girls. The reason behind doing this is the same as mentioned in the methods of pulse examination (Refer to Figure 2.1.3). With respect to illness, consider a hot disorder if the pulse looks black and thick, whereas yellowish-pale and thin is considered to be a cold disorder. The characteristics of a healthy pulse is red, clear, and of equal size. Apply the above-mentioned procedures to all the organs and parts of the body. Figure 2.3.1 shows the technique of examining a child's ear.

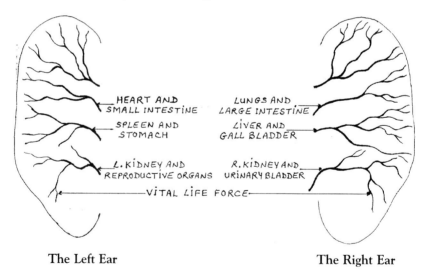

The Left Ear   The Right Ear

Figure 2.3.1: The Diagnostic Technique of Examining a Child's Ear

4. Examining the Breast Milk of a Mother

This is done to examine the illness of an infant from birth to one year old. The time of examination is in the morning when the sun rises from the east. To do this, fill one cupped handful of water in a clean bowl. Then pour a little bit of the mother's breast milk, squeezed from the right for a boy and the left for a girl, in a bowl of water for examination. This is because during the pregnancy, the right side of the womb is higher for boys, whereas the left side of the womb is higher for girls. Likewise, the breast milk comes first from the right to a boy and from the left to a girl.

Examining the Characteristics of Breast Milk:

Rlung disorder:	Tastes astringent and floats on the surface with bubbles
mKhris.Pa disorder:	Tastes sour and has yellowish tint
Bad.Kan disorder:	Tastes astringent and sour with a bluish tint, sticky, and sinks deep
Blood disorder:	Brownish tint

The balanced or healthy breast milk tastes sweet, is clear, and mixes properly with water.

5. Examining the Nose

The nostrils are doors of the lungs for inhaling and exhaling. The hairs inside them prevent foreign bodies, such as dust particles and pathogens. The nose is considered the flower of the lungs, therefore, we see nasal problems for people who have lung disorders. The size and capacity of the lungs can be inferred from the size of the nose, i.e. big or small. The nose captures smells because of nerve impulses. The nerve impulses are the function of branch *Rlung* called *rTsangs.Pa* (Kalachakra Tantra: perfectly moving *Rlung*). Regarding nasal sense consciousness, three conditions are required and their application is the same as previously mentioned in the eye examination.

Examining the Characteristics of a Nasal Disorder:

Chronic lung disease or *Rlung* disorder:	Sunken nostrils
Common cold:	Runny nose and irritations
Lung infection:	Stuffy nose with dryness of nasal openings
Pleural effusion:	Runny nose and redness at the tip of the nose

Stomach disorder:	Darkness at the tip of the nose
Chronic nasal disease:	Discharge of pus and sneezing
Bad.Kan disorder:	Stuffy nose and heaviness
Black lymph disorder:	Loss of smell, stuffy, and irritation
Nasal polyps:	Stuffy nose with thick watery discharge or bleeding, and swelling in and around nose

6. Examining the Tongue

The tongue is the site of experiencing Bad.Kan, which captures sweet, different tastes. It is also considered flower of the heart. Therefore, we see deep cracks in the center of the tongue for people who have heart Rlung disorder. The tongue capture tastes because of nerve impulses. The nerve impulses are the function of the branch Rlung called Lhas.sByin (Kalachakra Tantra: strongly moving Rlung). Regarding taste sense consciousness, three conditions are required and their application is the same as previously mentioned in the eye examination.

Examining the Characteristics of a Tongue Disorder:

Rlung disorder:	Red, coarse, dry with cracks or no cracks on it
Remnants of fever blown by Rlung:	Dry
Higher fever than Rlung:	Dry, inflexible, and tip of the tongue rolls back
Fever and Rlung of equal strength:	Dry and black
Empty fever:	Dry, coarse, and black in the center
mKhris.Pa disorder:	Thick and pale-yellowish coating with yellowish under the tongue
High mKhris.Pa fever:	Blackness in the center and tastes bitter
Bad.Kan disorder:	Pale, dull, smooth, and moist with sticky coating
High blood temperature:	Dry and red
Rlung and mKhris.Pa combined disorder:	Yellow, dry, and inflexible
Bad.Kan and Rlung combined disorder:	Pale, dry, and inflexible
Rlung spread complicated fever:	Pale, thick, and dull in color
Unripened fever:	Pale with tiny red pimples
Ripened fever:	Yellowish-pale with no pimples
High Bad.Kan sMug.Po fever:	Dry, inflexible, and tastes bitter
Heart fever:	Blackness on the tip of the tongue
Heart disorder:	Cracks or fissures in the center
High spleen fever:	Palish tongue with dark lips

Kidney disorder:	Parallel blackness on the two sides
High *Bad.Kan* in stomach and liver:	Fat-like thick coating
Bad.Kan sMug.Po:	Brownish with fissures
Poisoning:	Blackish with fissures
Tongue inflammation:	Swelling under the tongue with difficulty in speaking and eating
Acute tongue infection:	Swelling of the tongue fills whole mouth with a lot of saliva discharge and restriction in food movement
Enlarged epiglottis:	Swelling like cow's breast which prevents food and beverage from passing down and instead vomits up or comes out from the nostrils

The balanced or healthy tongue is red, smooth, moist, and flexible

7. *Examining the Lips*

The voice comes clear with the help of lips and is also considered a flower of the spleen. Therefore, when the spleen is sick, the signs appear on the lips.

Examining the Characteristics of a Lip Disorder:

Rlung disorder:	Hardening, cracks are dark, coarse, and painful
mKhris.Pa disorder:	Yellowish tint with little tolerance to hot things and appearance of mustard seed-like tiny pimples all over the lips from which oozes a lot of pus and fluid
Bad.Kan disorder:	Little tolerance to cold things with heaviness, swelling, and tiny pale pimples all over the lips
Tri-*Nyes.Pa* disorder:	Party-colored, oozes sticky and foul smelling fluid, and pus forms quick or slowly with or without swelling and pain
Blood disorder:	Red and bleeds

8. *Examining the Complexion*

The tone of the body's complexion depends on balanced *Nyes.Pa* (humor), vital life force (refer to number 13, Vital Life Force (*Bla*) Pulse in Part Two, Diagnosis by Pulse Examination), and particularly the vital fluid which abides in the heart. In *rGyud.bZhi*, this is called '*mDangs.*' It is formed from the essence of regenerative fluid, the seventh bodily constituent. Its vitality pervades the whole body, helps in enduring life, and provides bright complexion and physical radiance. Its vitality is reduced by mental suffering, fear, emaciation, debility, unhappiness, and poor complexion. Intake of milk and meat soups are considered remedies to promote the vital fluid (*mDangs*). The skin is also a common site where *mKhris.Pa* and *Rlung* abide together. The skin captures the tangible sensations such as roughness and softness because of nerve impulses. The nerve impulses are the functions of *Nor.rGyas* (Kalachakra Tantra: definitely moving *Rlung*). Regarding tangible sense consciousness, three conditions are required and their application is the same as previously mentioned in the eye examination.

Rlung disorder:	Dark
mKhris.Pa disorder:	Yellowish
Anemia or *Bad.Kan* disorder:	Pale
Tuberculosis or other chronic diseases:	Very poor
High impure blood:	Reddish-brown
Sign of pregnancy or stomach-spleen disorder:	Appearance of blemishes or black patches
Spleen disorder:	Pale and swollen lower lip

9. Examining the Sputum

Rlung disorder:	Expectorates pale and frothy or dark sputum
mKhris.Pa disorder:	Expectorates reddish-yellow with salty tasting sputum
Bad.Kan disorder:	Expectorates a lot of sticky and bluish tinted mucous
Pulmonary *Rlung* disorder:	Expectorates frothy phlegm in the early morning and evening with difficulty
Initial fluid accumulation in lungs:	Expectorates blood tinted frothy phlegm
Lungs fever:	Expectorates salty tasting or blood tinted sputum
Suppuration of lungs:	Expectorates bubbly sputum like the eyes of fish with pus
High fever:	Expectorates lot of dark and reddish-yellow sputum
Spread *Bad.Kan sMug.Po* disorder:	Expectorates brownish and blood-tinted sputum

Terminal disorder:	Expectorates a lot of dark and fleshy gruel-like sputum or accumulates them in the throat
Disturbed heart fever:	Expectorates pale and frothy sputum
Disturbed lung fever:	Expectorates reddish tint sputum
Disturbed liver fever:	Expectorates reddish-yellow tint sputum
Disturbed spleen fever:	Expectorates brownish-dark sputum
Disturbed kidney fever:	Expectorates brownish-red sputum
Disturbed vessel (blood) fever:	Expectorates intermittently with blood
Disturbed gall bladder fever:	Expectorates yellowish and clear sputum
Rlung combined disturbed fever:	Expectorates bluish and frothy sputum

10. Examining the Feces

Hot disorder:	Hard and dry
Cold disorder:	Thin with large quantity
Rlung disorder:	Watery and bubbly diarrhea with rumbling sound
mKhris.Pa disorder:	Reddish-yellow or greenish color or fleshy gruel-like diarrhea with little quantity, cramps, fetid and sinks deep in water
Bad.Kan disorder or cold–caused diarrhea:	Diarrhea with mucus and undigested food particles floating on the water
Liver fever:	Fleshy gruel-like diarrhea with reddish-brown in color
Dysentery:	Thin diarrhea with blood and mucus
High *mKhris.Pa* fever:	Very yellowish
Cold *mKhris.Pa* disorder: [5]	Pale and soft
Bad.Kan sMug.Po:	Brown and dry like deer's dung
Peptic or duodenal ulcer:	Dark
Hemorrhoids:	Blood stained stool or anal bleeding

11. Examining the Vomiting

Rlung disorder:	Dry heaves or frothy vomiting
mKhris.Pa disorder:	Yellow and bitter tasting vomiting

Indigestion or *Bad.Kan* disorder:	Vomits undigested food particles
Gastritis:	Sticky and sour water
Bad.Kan sMug.Po:	Fleshy gruel-like putrid blood vomiting
Bad.Kan and *Rlung* combined disorder:	Bubbly with mucus mixture

12. Examining the Blood

Under this topic, the characteristics of unhealthy and healthy blood are explained in order:

The Characteristics of Unhealthy Blood:

Unhealthy blood:	Bleeds strongly from the cuts (veins) of blood letting, thin, yellowish tint, and fetid, pale and sticky bubbles with appearance of scum-like mucus, pus, or bile
Mixture of healthy and unhealthy blood:	Red and dark blend blood

The Characteristics of Healthy Blood:

Blood of *Rlung* person:	Dark, coarse, and reddish-yellow tint bubbles
Blood of *mKhris.Pa* Person:	Yellowish tint, thin, and smells like pus with appearance of iron oxide on the surface
Blood of *Bad.Kan* person:	Reddish-pale, thick, smooth, and sticky
Blood of tri-*Nyes.Pa* balanced person:	Red, clear, like cinnabar or *Laccifer Lacca* (Red Lac) extracted in water and leaves no stain on clothes when washed

Although the examination of pulse and urine are the two most important diagnostic techniques from the touch and visual examination, the examination of a person's nature and secondary examinations are also important. Information concerning the disturbances of the organs and *Nyes.Pa* can also be gathered from secondary examinations. Therefore, it is also important to pay attention to them.

CHAPTER FOUR

DIAGNOSIS BY INTERROGATION

The interrogation is one of the three main diagnostic techniques in Tibetan medicine. It is very useful, informative, and instrumental in enabling the physician to see the clear picture of the patient's condition in conjunction with the visual and touch examination. Its main objectives are:

- to find the causative factors of an illness,
- to find the site of an illness, and
- to find the signs and symptoms.

1. Finding the Causative Factors of an Illness:

The questions pertaining to the causative factors are two main contributing factors of illnesses, the unwholesome food and beverage and improper behavior. The questions raised are:

- What kind of food and beverages has one taken?
- What kind of physical and mental behaviors has one gone through?

The answer the patient gives helps the physician in gathering clues for the clinical assessment as well as in determining the *Nyes.Pa* involved.

2. Finding the Site of an Illness:

Likewise, the questions pertaining to the site of an illness include asking about the pain and other abnormalities in the upper, middle, and lower part of the body or internal and external organs in understanding the main site affected by the illness. This enables the physician to determine the general pathways or passages of disorders. See Branch 3: General Passages of *Nyes.Pa* in Part One, Chapter Three: The Basis of Normal and Abnormal Body.

3. Finding the Signs and Symptoms:

Finally, the questions pertaining to the manifestation of signs and symptoms associated with the specific disorders are asked in order to correlate them with the previously mentioned causative factors and the site of an illness. The questions raised here may cover the degrees of body aches, temperature, sleeping and digestion, etc., with a wide range of topics. This is especially important for a physician in understanding and differentiating each and every disease correctly. The interrogation is an art which may actually become instrumental in raising confidence and trust if used correctly and to the point.

Part Three
Case History

THE TIBETAN MEDICINE
AND THE BDORT

Tenzing Dakpa, M.D.
Men-Tsee-Khang (Tibetan Medical and Astrological Institute
of H. H. the Dalai Lama)
Gangchen Kyishong, Dharamsala, India

Yasuhiro Shimotsuura M.D., F.I.C.A.E.
Vice President, Japan Bi-Digital O-Ring Test;
O-Ring Test Life Science Research Institute and Shimotsuura Clinic,
Kurume, Fukuoka, Japan

Shigeharu Fukuda Ph.D. and Takashi Shibuya
Amase Institute of Hayashibara Biochemical Laboratories, Inc.
Okayama, Japan

Yoshiaki Omura, Sc.D., F.A.C.A., F.I.C.A.E.
Adjunct Professor of Preventive Medicine, New York Medical College;
Professor of Non-Orthodox Medicine,
Ukrainian National Medical University, Kiev, Ukraine;
Director, Heart Disease Research Foundation;
President, International College of Acupuncture & Electro-Therapeutics,
New York

ABSTRACT

The practice of Tibetan pulse and urine examination appears simple, yet they are very complex diagnostic techniques. An in-depth study of the two subjects is essential for building the skills necessary for a correct diagnosis.

For instance, the pulse is like a messenger who gives the messages from the patient's abnormal site to a physician. These messages, like weak or strong pulse beats, are transmitted to the radial artery by *Rlung* (pronounced as "loong" and has nothing to do with "lung"). *Rlung* is an energy that governs the functions of the nervous system, respiration, and cardiovascular system—most of the physical functions including mental. Messages, like impulses, are picked up at the radial artery by a physician's index, middle, and ring fingers of both hands.

The best time for examining the pulse is in the morning when a patient has not eaten or drunk anything or engaged in physical exertion. The pulse is examined on the radial artery of the patient's left and right wrist by measuring the width of the patient's distal phalanx of thumb from the first crease of the wrist. The amounts of pressure applied on the patient's radial arteries are:

Index fingers:	Pressed lightly to feel the skin
Middle fingers:	Pressed moderately to feel flesh
Ring fingers:	Pressed strongly to feel bone

The left wrist of a male patient is examined first, whereas the right wrist is examined first for a female. Then the opposite wrists are examined. For a male patient, the physician examines the condition of the heart, small intestine, spleen, stomach, left kidney, and reproductive organs on the left radial artery, and examines the lungs, large intestine, liver, gall bladder, right kidney, and urinary bladder on the right radial artery. Note that for females the organs beneath the index fingers are reversed from those of males. This differentiation is made because of the gender. Abnormalities from the organs or upper, middle, or lower parts of the body are determined under the index, middle, and ring fingers of both hands and from the following pulse characteristics of imbalanced *Rlung*, *mKhris.Pa*, and *Bad.Kan*.

Disorders	Pulse Characteristics
Rlung disorder:	Thick-like sack distended by air, floats on the surface, and is empty when pressed. There is a pause between pulse beats at indefinite pulse counts.
mKhris.Pa disorder:	Fast, prominent, thin, and taut like rolled horse tail, and does not halt beat when pressed
Bad.Kan disorder:	Unclear, deeply sunken, weak, and slow

Refer to Figure 3.1.1, which shows the fingers and hands of a doctor defining the pulse examination points and their corresponding body parts.

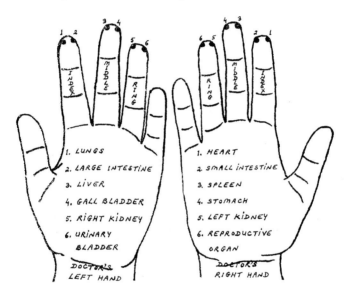

Figure 3.1.1: A Doctor's Hands and the Corresponding Examination Sites

The urine is like a mirror that reflects the features of disorders. Since it is an end product of the body fluid, it carries the features of disorders. The features like color, vapor, and bubbles, etc., are examined for a diagnosis.

The examination of the patient's first morning mid-stream urine is performed at three different temperatures: (1) warm, (2) lukewarm, and (3) cold. The physician examines the color, vapor, odor, and bubbles for the just-voided urine. The sediments and scum are examined when the urine is lukewarm. Finally, the time of urine's change, modes of change, and the post-change qualities are examined when the urine is cooled.

All of those characteristics are examined from the same urine and the examination of the urine is performed in daylight to determine clearly the intensity of color, vapor, and sediments of the urine. For examination, the urine is poured into a cup that is white on the inside to prevent discoloration of the urine. The container must be clean and devoid of contamination. The urine is stirred with sticks to facilitate observation of changes.

Like the pulse, the abnormalities of imbalanced *Rlung*, *mKhris.Pa*, and *Bad.Kan* are determined from the following characteristics of urine. Refer to Figure 3.1.2, which shows the mode of examining the urine.

Disorders	Urine Characteristics
Rlung disorder:	Bluish and thin like spring water with large bubbles when stirred
mKhris.Pa disorder:	Yellowish-red with lots of steam, fetid, and quickly disappearing tiny bubbles when stirred
Bad.Kan disorder:	Whitish with light odor and vapor, and saliva-like bubbles when stirred

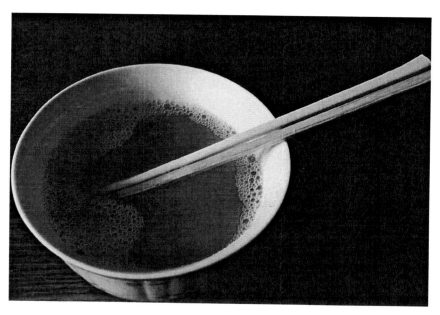

Figure 3.1.2: The Mode of Examining the Urine

There are also certain prerequisite conditions to be observed both by the patient and the physician. For instance, the night before the examination, the patient should refrain from drinking excessive strong tea, buttermilk, or alcohol and taking vitamins to avoid altering the characteristics and discoloration of the urine sample. Refer to prerequisite conditions of Part Two, Chapter Two, and the Diagnosis by Urine Examination. Both the patient and the physician must refrain from physical and mental stress and have a good night's rest to avoid the disturbances in the nature of the illness and the misdiagnosis, respectively.

The techniques of pulse and urine examination have been practiced for centuries and are unique to Tibetan medicine. The "Bi-Digital O-Ring Test" as explained and practiced by Professor Yoshiaki Omura and his associate Professor Yasuhiro Shimotsuura is a simple, non-invasive, safe, and quick new diagnostic method. The application of the BDORT method may have a significant role in the future. Figure 3.1.3 shows the author with Professor Yasuhiro Shimotsuura and his associates at the O-Ring Test Life Science Research Institute and Shimotsuura Clinic in Kurume, Fukuoka, Japan (seated in the front row from extreme left are Professor Yasuhiro Shimotsuura, author, Dr. Dawa, Mrs. Yasuko Shimotsuura, Dr. Nishimura, and Mr. Oki and Mrs. Takeuchi, standing second and fifth in the second row from left).

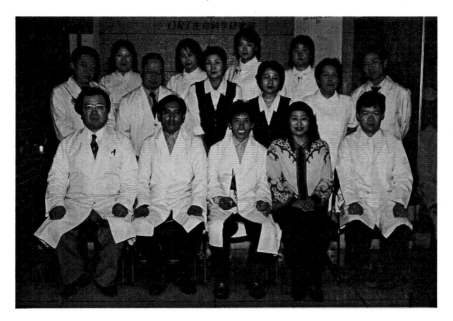

Figure 3.1.3: Author with Professor Shimotsuura and his Associates

BDORT and Professor Omura

The Bi-Digital O-Ring Test is a simple, non-invasive, safe, and quick new diagnostic method developed by Professor Yoshiaki Omura in the early 1970s. According to him, physicians in the U.S.A., Scandinavian countries, Germany, Belgium, England, Japan, China, Korea, and Venezuela have been using this technique since the early 1980s. He holds, every year, the Annual International Symposium on Acupuncture, Electro-Therapeutics and Bi-Digital O-Ring Test at Columbia University in October and three days of seminar and workshops on Acupuncture and Electro-Therapeutics in Clinical Practice every month except in July, August, and October in New York City. He also sees patients during the seminar and workshop. He is President of the International College of Acupuncture and Electro-Therapeutics as well as Editor-in-Chief and Founder of *Acupuncture and Electro-Therapeutics Research, The International Journal*. He works very hard spreading the message of BDORT to serve more people. He is also a physician, educator, electrical engineer, and experimental physicist.

O-Ring Test Life Science Research Institute and Shimotsuura Hospital

The O-Ring Test Life Science Research Institute and Shimotsuura Hospital is in Kurume, Fukuoka, Japan. Professor Yasuhiro Shimotsuura, M.D., F.I.C.A.E., is Chief Medical Officer and Director of the O-Ring Test Life Science Research Institute and Shimotsuura Hospital and Vice President of the Japan Bi-Digital O-Ring Test Medical Association. He is also the most outstanding student of Professor Yoshiaki Omura. He has been successfully practicing the Bi-Digital O-Ring Test developed by Professor Omura for many years. During my two-month stay in Kurume, Japan, in 2000, I witnessed Professor Shimotsuura seeing patients suffering from all sorts of problems, including cancer. The readers will see the images drawn on the patients' body by Professor Shimotsuura using an O-Ring technique with the help of a nurse, Mrs. Takeuchi, as a third person in the following case histories. He and his wife, Mrs. Yasuko Shimotsuura, are kind-hearted, jovial, and good humored people. I noticed their associates and patients love and respect them. I also began to feel very close to all of them as well as to the Amase Institute of Hayashibara Biochemical Laboratories in Okayama, Japan, and to its President, Mr. Ken Hayashibara. I owe them for their kindness and support for the following case histories.

The preceding conditions about the patients' case presentation are:
1. The following patients were seen at the O-Ring Test Life Science Research Institute and Shimotsuura Clinic in Kurume, Japan from September 25 to October 3, 2000. The permission was granted by Professor Yasuhiro Shimotsuura, M.D., F.I.C.A.E.
2. I was seeing them for the first time and was told nothing about the patients' condition. Since most of the patients did not speak English, Mr. Oki (the secretary to Professor Shimotsuura) translated for us.
3. Mr. Oki was also taking notes of each patient I saw as well as grading of the BDORT.
4. The image of finger placement on the patients' right and left wrists were drawn after placing my index, middle, and ring fingers of both hands.
5. Those small black rounds on either side of the doctor's finger represent pulse examination points and their corresponding body parts. The upper, middle, and lower parts of the body are examined under the doctor's index, middle, and ring fingers of both hands.

116

6. The grades of O-Ring tests were made with the help of my colleague, Dr. Dawa, holding a metal rod in his left hand at the site of each organ representation on the patients' radial arteries. I used his thumb and ring finger of his right hand for this test.

7. The examinations of the patients' urine were done by shaking a transparent bottle as well as stirring the urine in a paper cup with chopsticks.

8. The findings of each patient's health problems were based on pulse and urine examination.

9. Later, Professor Yasuhiro Shimotsuura confirmed each patient's health problems from their respective files as well as provided their medical reports. He also wrote the name of the diseases on the patient's palms.

10. Finally, I am pleased to inform here that my findings matched Professor Yasuhiro Shimotsuura's diagnosis. I think this was due to my fervent prayer to the Medicine Buddha as well as the full concentration I paid on each patient's health conditions during the examination. Otherwise I would not have succeeded in finding the problems of some patients.

ACTUAL CASE PRESENTATION

Patient no. 1
Sex: Female
Age: 50
Date: September 25, 2000

The findings of the pulse examination:
(1) A hypertension was felt from the pulse beats i.e., thick, full, and overflowing under the upper side of the right and left index fingers, the heart and lungs. They indicate *Rlung* and blood combined disorder.
(2) An abnormality in the left kidney was felt from the pulse beats i.e., weak, sunken, and unclear under the upper side of the right ring finger and the left kidney. They indicate a *Bad.Kan* disorder.

Refer to Figure 3.1.4 which shows a patient's hand and the corresponding examination sites.

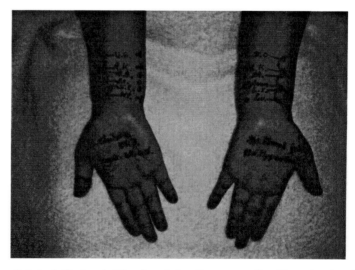

Figure 3.1.4: A Patient's Hand and the Corresponding Examination Sites

The findings of the urine examination:

(1) A cold *Rlung* disorder was noted from the clear and transparent urine.

(2) A renal failure was suspected from the settling of whitish sediments at the bottom of the container. Such urine characteristics indicate a *Bad.Kan* disorder.

Refer to Figure 3.1.5, which shows a patient's urine.

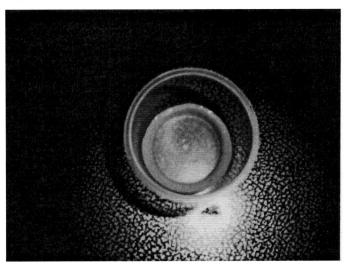

Figure 3.1.5: A Patient's Urine

Conclusion: A cold disorder.

The information provided from the patient's file is:

(1) Hypertension (BP: 188-108 mmHg)

(2) Renal failure

BUN (Blood urea nitrogen)

Abnormal: 30.7 mg/dl   (Normal range: 8-20)

Cr (Creatinin)

Abnormal: 11.15 mg/dl   (Normal range: 0.40-0.80)

Peritonin dialysis—4 times a day at home.

• • •

Patient no. 2

Sex: Female

Age: 73

Date: September 25, 2000

The findings of the pulse examination:

(1) A hypertension was felt from the pulse beats i.e., thick, superficial, and empty under the upper side of the right and left index fingers, the heart and lungs. They indicate *Rlung* disorder.

(2) Suspected myocardial infarction, poor blood circulation, and numbness and tingling sensation in the hands from the pulse beat i.e., weak under the upper side of the left index finger, and the heart. The weak pulse indicates a *Bad.Kan* disorder.

Refer to Figure 3.1.6, which shows a patient's hand and the corresponding examination sites.

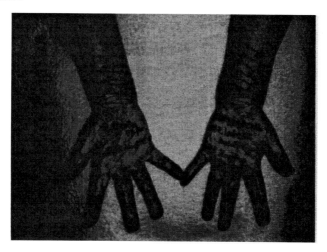

Figure 3.1.6: A Patient's Hand and the Corresponding Examination Sites

The findings of the urine examination:

(1) *Rlung* and *Bad.Kan* combined cold disorder was noted from the clear, transparent, and whitish-yellow urine that was frothy with many bubbles on the edge of the urine.

(2) The color of the urine in a cup is altered by the reflection of light from above.

Refer to Figure 3.1.7, which shows a patient's urine.
Insert Figure 3.1.7 Here

Figure 3.1.7: A Patient's Urine

Conclusion: A cold disorder.
The information provided from the patient's file is:
(1) Hypertension (BP: 184-104 mmHg)
(2) Ischemic heart disease

(3) Tingling sensation in the hands

Cholesterol

Abnormal: 248 mg/dl   (Normal range: 130-220)

Tryglycerides (TG)

Abnormal: 214 mg/dl   (Normal range: 40-150)

Refer to Figure 3.1.8 for an O-Ring image of a patient's heart. The image was drawn by Professor Shimotsuura using an O-Ring technique with the help of a nurse, Takeuchi, as a third person.

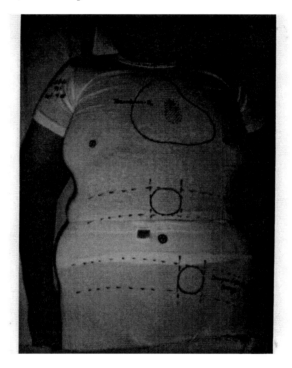

Figure 3.1.8: An O-Ring Image of a Patient's Heart

•••

Patient no. 3

Sex: Male

Age: 61

Date: September 26, 2000

The findings of the pulse examination:

(1) The stomach malfunction was felt from the pulse beats i.e., weak and thin under the lower side of the right middle finger, the stomach. They indicate a

121

chronic indigestion.

(2) An abnormality in the upper part of the small intestine was suspected from the pulse beats i.e., overflowing, taut, and thin under the lower side of the right index finger, the small intestine. They indicate a blood and *mKhris.Pa* disorder.

(3) An abnormality in the colon was felt from the pulse beats i.e., weak and thin under the lower side of the left index finger, the large intestine. They also indicate a chronic indigestion as mentioned above.

(4) An occasional low back problem was noted from the pulse beats i.e., weak and sunken under the upper side of the right and left ring fingers, the kidneys. They indicate a *Bad.Kan* disorder.

Refer to Figure 3.1.9, which shows a patient's hand and the corresponding examination sites.

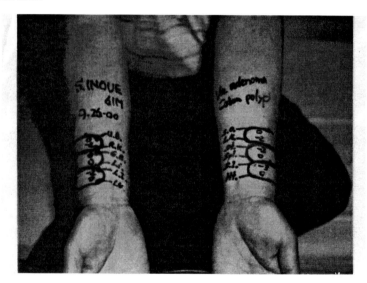

Figure 3.1.9: A Patient's Hand and the Corresponding Examination Sites

The findings of the urine examination:
(1) An inflammation was noted from the crackling sounds during the disappearance of bubbles in the urine.
(2) A *Bad.Kan* disorder was noted from the light sediments in the urine.

Refer to Figures 3.1.10, which shows a patient's urine

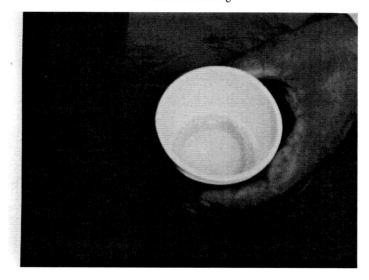

Figure 3.1.10: A Patient's Urine

Conclusion: The *Bad.Kan* and *mKhris.Pa* combined gastrointestinal malfunction with an abnormality in the pancreas was suspected from both the pulse and urine examination. The low back problem was not a major concern for the patient.

The information provided from the patient's file is:
(1) Pancreatic head or ampulla of Vater adenoma
(2) Colon polyp

		2000/01/06		2000/04/04		2000/06/01		2000/08/01		2000/09/01	
HbA1	6.0~8.0	H	9.0	H	9.2	H	9.1	H	9.2	H	8.4
HbA1C	4.3~5.8	H	7.0	H	7.1	H	7.1	H	7.2	H	6.5

2000/01/06	190 CEA (EIA)	H	5.7	(Normal range < 5.0)
2000/06/22	170 CEA (EIA)		5.0	(Normal range <5.0)
	220 CA 19-9 (EIA)		3.4	(Normal range < 37)
2000/08/01	170 CEA (EIA)	H	5.3	(Normal range < 5.0)
2000/09/07	170 CEA (EIA)		5.0	(Normal range < 5.0)

Refer to Figures 3.1.11 and 3.1.12 for endoscopic pictures of a pancreatic head and an O-Ring image of a pancreas and other organs, respectively. The image was drawn by Professor Shimotsuura using an O-Ring technique with the help of a nurse, Takeuchi, as a third person.

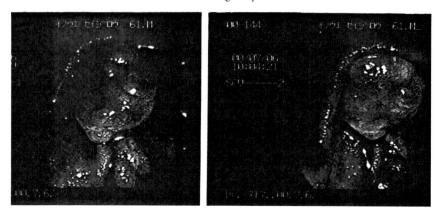

Figure 3.1.11: Endoscopic Pictures of Pancreatic Head

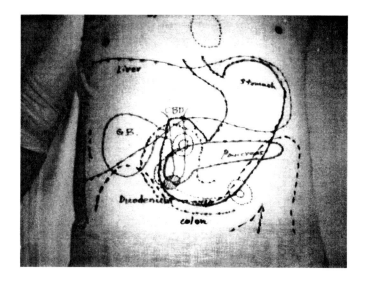

Figure 3.1.12: An O-Ring Image of a Patient's Pancreas and other Organs

•   •   •

Patient no. 4
Sex: Female
Age: 59
Date: September 26, 2000

The findings of the pulse examination:
(1) An injury or surgery to the uterus or ovary was suspected from the pulse

beats i.e., weak and unclear under the lower side of the right ring finger, the reproductive organ. Such pulse beats also indicate the removal of the respective organ.

(2) The ringing in ears were felt from the pulse beats i.e., floating and empty under the upper side of the right and left ring fingers, the kidneys. They also indicate *Rlung* disorder.

Refer to Figure 3.1.13, which shows a patient's hands and the corresponding examination sites.

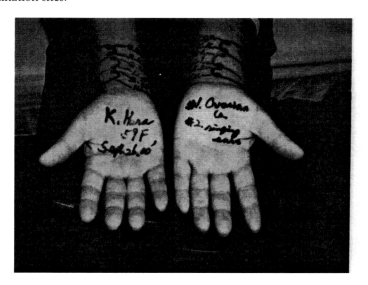

Figure 3.1.13: A Patient's Hand and the Corresponding Examination Sites

The findings of the urine examination:
(1) An infection was suspected from the dark colored urine.
(2) *Rlung* and *Bad.Kan* combined disorder was noted from the air-filled and saliva-like bubbles in the urine.

Refer to Figure 3.1.14 which shows a patient's urine.

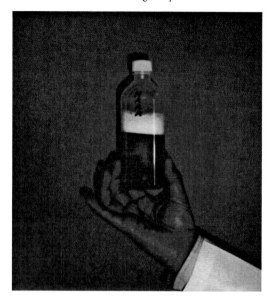

Figure 3.1.14: A Patient's Urine

Conclusion: *Rlung* and *Bad.Kan* combined cold disorder.

The information provided from the patient's file is:
(1) Ringing in ears
(2) Ovarian cancer (right or left ovary has been removed)
(3) Peritonitis carcinomatosa
(4) The patient was on treatment for recurrent cancer

2000/08/03	CA 19-9 (EIA)		3.6	(Normal range <37)
2000/08/03	CA 125 (RIA)	H	45.5	(Normal range <35)

Refer to Figures 3.1.15, 3.1.16, and 3.1.17 for peritonitis carcinomatosa pictures, echosonographies of ovarian cancer, and an O-Ring image of a womb and liver, respectively. The image was drawn by Professor Shimotsuura using an O-Ring technique with the help of a nurse, Takeuchi, as a third person.

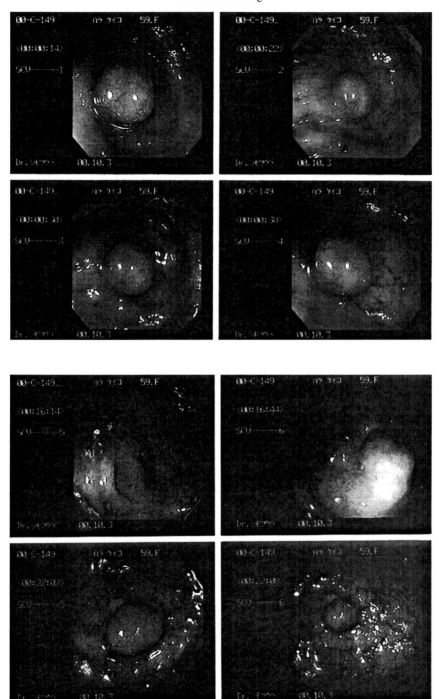

Figure 3.1.15: Peritonitis Carcinomatosa

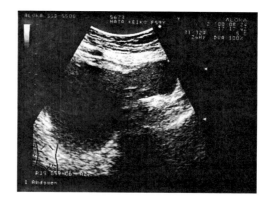

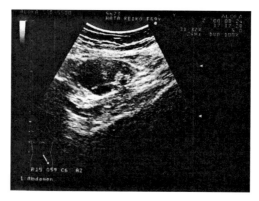

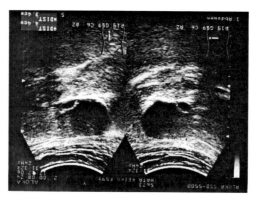

Figure 3.1.16: Echosonographies of ovarian cancer

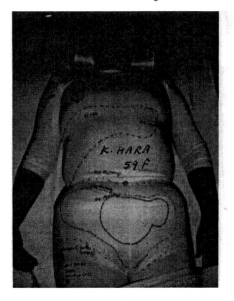

Figure 3.1.17: An O-Ring Image of a Womb and a Liver

. . .

Patient no. 5
Sex: Female
Age: 58
Date: September 26, 2000

The findings of the pulse examination:

(1) A mental stress and the elevation of blood pressure were felt from the pulse beats i.e., superficial and empty under the upper side of the right and left index fingers, the heart, and lungs. They indicate *Rlung* disorder.

(2) An injury or surgery to the right side of the abdomen was felt from the pulse beats i.e., weak and unclear under the lower side of the right and left index fingers, the small and large intestine. Such pulse beats also indicate a removal of the organ.

Refer to Figure 3.1.18, which shows a patient's hand and the corresponding examination sites.

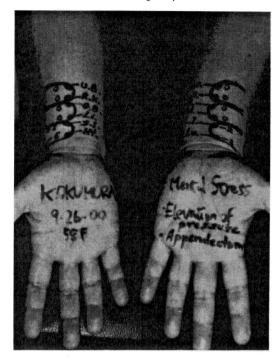

Figure 3.1.18: A Patient's Hand and the Corresponding Examination Sites

Conclusion: *Rlung* disorder

The information provided from the patient's file is:
(1) Mental stress
(2) Elevation of blood pressure
(3) Appendectomy

Refer to Figure 3.1.19 for an O-Ring image of a patient's abdomen. The image was drawn by Professor Shimotsuura using an O-Ring technique with the help of a nurse, Takeuchi, as a third person.

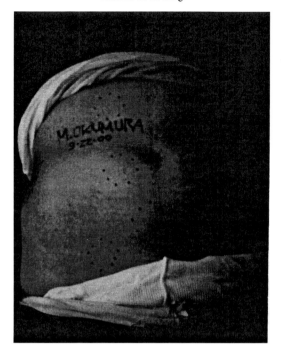

Figure 3.1.19: An O-Ring Image of a Patient's Abdomen

• • •

Patient no. 6
Sex: Female
Age: 75
Date: September 26, 2000

The findings of the pulse examination:
(1) I examined this patient on her third visit to the clinic. She was receiving treatment for tuberculosis.
(2) A pain in the lower back was felt from the pulse beats, i.e., empty and slow under the upper side of the right and left ring fingers, the kidneys. They in turn indicate *Rlung* and *Bad.Kan* disorders.

Refer to Figure 3.1.20 which shows a patient's hand and the corresponding examination sites.

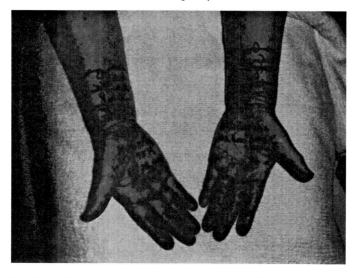

Figure 3.1.20: A Patient's Hand and the Corresponding Examination Sites

The findings of the urine examination:
(1) *Rlung* disorder was noted from the clear, transparent, and air-filled large bubbles.
(2) A *Bad.Kan* disorder was felt from the stable and saliva-like bubbles on the edges of the container.
(3) The color of the urine in a paper cup was altered by the light from above.

Refer to Figure 3.1.21, which show a patient's urine. Note the difference of color of the same urine in a transparent bottle and a paper cup. The color of urine in a paper cup was altered by the light from above.

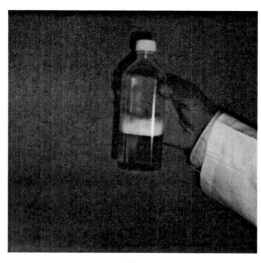

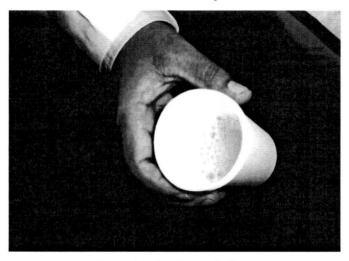

Figure 3.1.21: Patient's Urine

Conclusion: *Rlung* and *Bad.Kan* combined cold disorder.

The information provided from the patient's file is:
(1) Tuberculosis
(2) Low back pain

Refer to Figure 3.1.22 for an O-Ring image of a patient's right lung. The image was drawn by Professor Shimotsuura using an O-Ring technique with the help of a nurse, Takeuchi, as a third person. He also tested the effect of rose geranium against tuberculosis using the same technique mentioned above. The result that came was highly positive (+ 4).

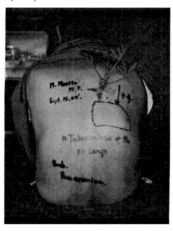

Figure 3.1.22: An O-Ring Image of a Patient's Right Lung

Patient no. 7
Sex: Female
Age: 46
Date: September 27, 2000

The findings of the pulse examination:
(1) The following problems were felt from the pulse beats i.e., thick and protruding under the lower side of the right ring finger, the reproductive organ. An abnormal menstruation with pain in the lower abdomen and lower back A pain or swelling in the breast
The pulse beats mentioned above indicate *Rlung* and blood disorder.
(2) An abnormality in the liver was suspected from the pulse beat i.e., protruding under the upper side of the left middle finger, the liver. This also indicates a blood disorder.
(3) A renal problem was felt from the pulse beats i.e., protruding yet sunken under the upper side of the right ring finger, the left kidney. They indicate a blood and *Bad.Kan* disorder.
(4) An abnormality in the stomach was felt from the pulse beat i.e., sunken under the lower side of the right middle finger, the stomach. The sunken pulse beat indicates a *Bad.Kan* disorder.

Refer to Figure 3.1.23, which shows a patient's hand and the corresponding examination sites.

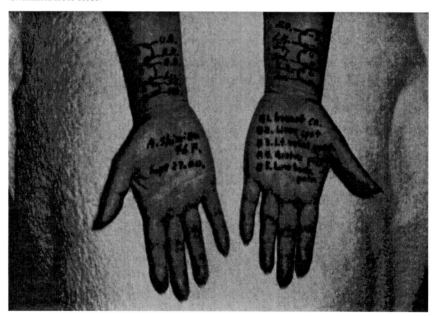

Figure 3.1.23: A Patient's Hand and the Corresponding Examination Sites

Conclusion: *Rlung*, blood, and *Bad.Kan* combined disorder.

The information provided from the patient's file is:
(1) Breast cancer
(2) Liver cyst
(3) Left renal cyst
(4) Gastric polyps
(5) Low back pain

Refer to Figure 3.1.24 for an O-Ring image of a patient's stomach and other organs. The image was drawn by Professor Shimotsuura using an O-Ring technique with the help of a nurse, Takeuchi, as a third person.

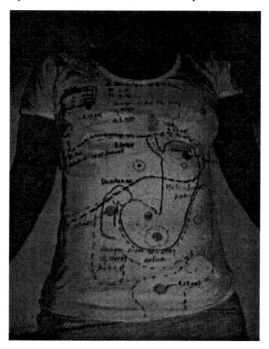

Figure 3.1.24: An O-Ring Image of a Patient's Stomach and other Organs

• • •

Patient no. 8
Sex: Male
Age: 78
Date: September 27, 2000

The findings of the pulse examination:

(1) A problem in the prostate, lower back, and kidneys was felt from the pulse beats, i.e., empty and slow under the upper side of the right and left ring fingers (kidneys) and lower side of the right ring finger (reproductive organ). They indicate *Rlung* and *Bad.Kan* disorders.

(2) A problem in the stomach was felt from the pulse beats, i.e., weak and slow under the lower side of the right middle finger, the stomach. They indicate a *Bad.Kan* disorder.

(3) A chest congestion and respiratory problem were felt from the pulse beats, i.e., weak and empty under the upper the side of the left index finger, the lungs. They indicate a *Bad.Kan* and *Rlung* disorder.

Refer to Figure 3.1.25 which shows a patient's hand and the corresponding examination sites.

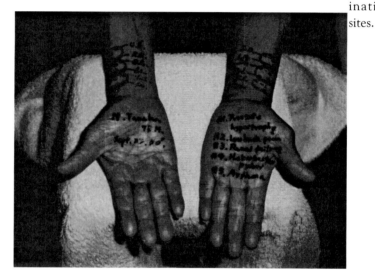

Figure 3.1.25: A Patient's Hand and the Corresponding Examination Sites

The findings of the urine examination:

(1) A *Bad.Kan* disorder was noted from the stable and saliva-like frothy bubbles on the surface of the urine.

(1) *Rlung* disorder was noted from the clear, transparent, and light sediments in the urine.

Refer to Figure 3.1.26 which shows a patient's urine.

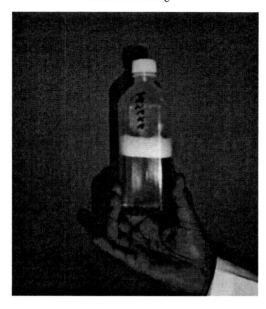

Figure 3.1.26: A Patient's Urine

Conclusion: *Rlung* and *Bad.Kan* combined cold disorder.

The information provided from the patient's file is:
(1) Prostate hypertrophy
(2) Low back pain
(3) Renal failure
(4) Helicobacter pylori
(5) Asthma

2000/02/17	PSA (IRMA)	H	7.6	(Normal range <4.0)
2000/03/10	PSA (IRMA)	H	7.6	(Normal range <4.0)
2000/04/03	PSA (IRMA)	H	7.6	(Normal range <4.0)
2000/05/15	PSA	H	5.7	(Normal range <4.0)
2000/06/14	PSA	H	6.0	(Normal range <4.0)
2000/07/18	PSA	H	6.6	(Normal range <4.0)
2000/08/17	PSA	H	6.1	(Normal range <4.0)

Refer to Figures 3.1.27 and 3.1.28 for echosonographies of a patient's abdomen and O-Ring images of prostate and lower back, respectively. The images were drawn by Professor Shimotsuura using an O-Ring technique with the help of a nurse, Takeuchi, as a third person.

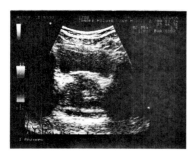
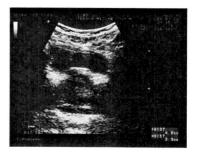
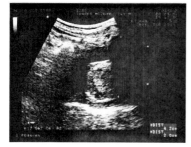
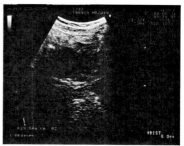
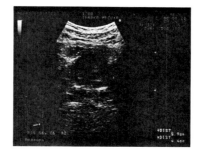

Figure 3.1.27: Echosonographies of Patient's Abdomen

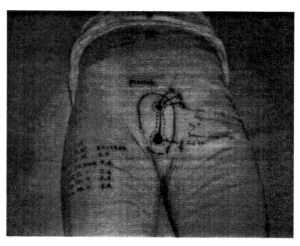

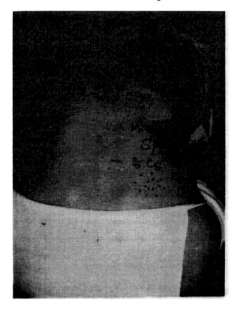

Figure 3.1.28: O-Ring Images of Prostate and Lower Back

• • •

Patient no. 9
Sex: Female
Age: 58
Date: September 27, 2000

The findings of the pulse examination:
(1) A malfunction of the gastrointestinal system was felt from the pulse beats i.e., thin and declining under the lower side of the right middle and index fingers (stomach and small intestine) and lower side of the left index finger (large intestine). They indicate a chronic cold conditioned *Bad.Kan sMug.Po.*

Refer to Figure 3.1.29 which shows a patient's hand and the corresponding examination sites.

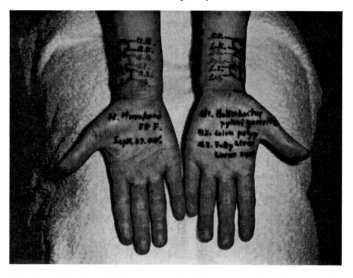

Figure 3.1.29: A Patient's Hand and the Corresponding Examination Sites

Conclusion: A chronic cold disorder.

The information provided from the patient's file is:
(1) Helicobacter pyroli gastritis
(2) Colon polyps
(3) Fatty liver and liver cyst

• • •

Patient no. 10
Sex: Female
Age: 62
Date: September 29, 2000

The findings of the pulse examination:
(1) A hypertension was felt from the pulse beat, i.e., protruding under the upper side of the right and left index fingers, the heart and lungs. The protruding pulse beat indicates a blood disorder.
(2) A renal dysfunction was felt from the pulse beats, i.e., protruding yet weak and sunken under the upper side of the right and left ring fingers, the kidneys. They indicate a blood and *Bad.Kan* combined disorders.
(3) Suspected a problem in the liver, gall bladder, and stomach from the pulse beats, i.e., weak and sunken under the upper and lower side of the left middle finger (liver and gall bladder), and lower side of the right middle finger (stomach). They indicate a *Bad.Kan* disorder.

140

Refer to Figure 3.1.30 which shows a patient's hand and the corresponding examination sites.

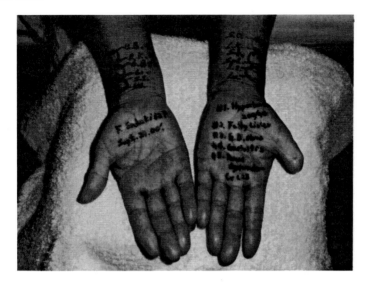

Figure 3.1.30: A Patient's Hand and the Corresponding Examination Sites

Conclusion: A blood and *Bad.Kan* combined disorder.

The information provided from the patient's file is:
(1) Hypertension (BP: 200-94 mmHg)
(2) Fatty liver
(3) Gallbladder stone
(4) Gastritis
(5) Renal dysfunction
(6) Cr (Creatinin) 1.23

• • •

Patient no. 11
Sex: Male
Age: 50
Date: September 29, 2000

The findings of the pulse examination:
(1) A problem in the gastrointestinal system was felt from the pulse beat i.e., weak under the lower side of the right and left index fingers (small and large intestine), and lower side of the right middle finger (stomach). The weak pulse beat indicates a *Bad.Kan* disorder.

141

(2) A problem in the liver was felt from the pulse beats i.e., firm and stronger under the upper side of the left middle finger, the liver. They indicate a blood and *mKhris.Pa* disorder.

(3) Noted a weak and strong pulse beat under the right (left radial artery) and left (right radial artery) fingers, respectively.

Refer to Figure 3.1.31, which shows a patient's hand and the corresponding examination sites.

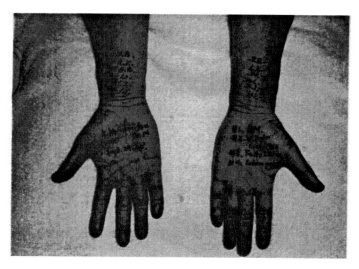

Figure 3.1.31: A Patient's Hand and the Corresponding Examination Sites

The findings of the urine examination:
(1) *Rlung* disorder was noted from the clear, transparent, and light sediments in the urine.
(2) A *Bad.Kan* disorder was noted from the stable and saliva-like frothy bubbles on the surface of the urine.

Refer to Figure 3.1.32 which shows a patient's urine.

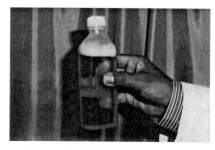

Figure 3.1.32: A Patient's Urine

Conclusion: A cold conditioned *Bad.Kan sMug.Po.*

The information provided from the patient's file is:
(1) Helicobacter pylori gastritis
(2) Fatty liver
(3) Colon polyps
(4) Diabetes mellitus

Refer to Figure 3.1.33 for an O-Ring image of a patient's stomach and other organs. The image was drawn by Professor Shimotsuura using an O-Ring technique with the help of a nurse, Takeuchi, as a third person.

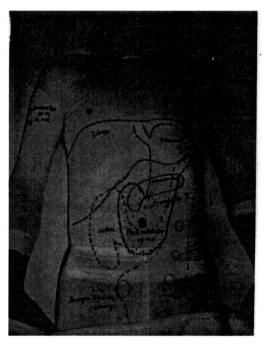

Figure 3.1.33: An O-Ring Image of a Patient's Stomach and other Organs

•　•　•

Patient no. 12
Sex: Female
Age: 76
Date: October 3, 2000

The findings of the pulse examination:
(1) A hypertension was felt from the pulse beats, i.e., superficial and empty

143

under the upper side of the right and left index fingers, the heart and lungs. They indicate *Rlung* disorder.

(2) A problem in the gall bladder and kidneys was felt from the pulse beats i.e., declining and slow under the lower side of the left middle finger (gall bladder), and upper side of the right and left ring fingers, the kidneys. They indicate a *Bad.Kan* disorder.

Refer to Figure 3.1.34 which shows a patient's hand and the corresponding examination sites.

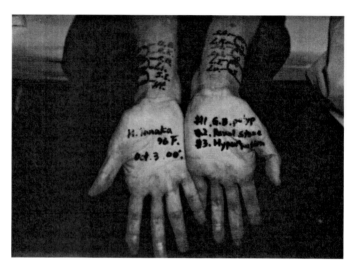

Figure 3.1.34: A Patient's Hand and the Corresponding Examination Sites

Conclusion: *Rlung* and *Bad.Kan* combined cold disorder.

The information provided from the patient's file is:
(1) Hypertension
(2) Gall bladder polyp
(3) Renal stone

Refer to Figure 3.1.35 for an echosonography of a patient's gall bladder.

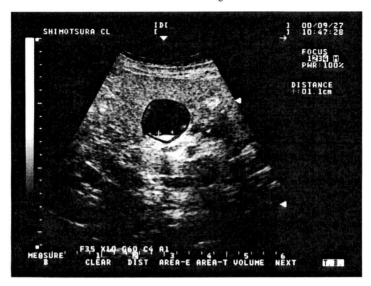

Figure 3.1.35: An Echosonography of a Patient's Gallbladder

NOTES

Introduction

1. The Tibetan medical history references to Galenos, once thought to refer to the Galen, known to Western medical historians as the founder of experimental physiology, are now thought to refer to a physician trained in the tradition of Galen (i.e., a follower of Galen). A clear explication was not found in the Tibetan medical texts.

Chapter One

1. It is traditional to begin a Sanskrit title to any major Tibetan text in order to make it more authentic and valuable. It is also believed to be auspicious to use Sanskrit, since Buddha himself taught in that language. Even to this day it is used for various book titles.
2. "gSang.Ba Man.Ngag Gi rGyud" implies that this medical tradition is an esoteric teaching whose genuine knowledge and practice leads one directly to the state of ultimate bliss or nirvana. In fact, this is one of the unbroken lineage-oriented medical teachings. A practitioner must be well prepared and formally initiated by the master, or else he or she may face various obstacles in life. Maintaining a high spiritual life and generating genuine compassion and love for the patient is necessary in order to practice this medical teaching.
3. It also means heart. Heart is one of the main organs of our body, which is considered the site of consciousness as well as energies and is attributed to emotions, feelings, thoughts and personality, etc. It also indicates rGyud.bZhi (Four Tantras) as the heart of Tibetan medicine.
4. The great trio of Ayurveda, the Caraka, Sushruta, and Vagbhata classifies the eight branches as follows:

Kaya cikitsa	Internal medicine
Salya tantra	Surgery
Salakya tantra	Treatment of diseases of head and neck including senses

146

Bhuta vidya	Psychotherapy
Agada tantra	Toxicology
Bala roga	Pediatrics
Rasayana tantra	Science of rejuvenation
Vajikarana tantra	Science of aphrodisiacs

5. Sogyal Rinpoche in his book *The Tibetan Book of Living and Dying*, says: In Tibetan the word for body is Lu which means "something you leave behind," like baggage. The medical connotation is to depend upon. Due to the interdependence upon each of the energies, and bodily constituents and excretions, the body forms, endures and disintegrates; and because they are, the root of this process is called *Lus* "the body." It consists of embryology, anatomy, physiology, pathology, internal disorders, and pharmacology, etc.

6. This refers to a wide range of forces and emotions, which are normally beyond conscious control, and all of them prevent well-being of body, speech, and mind and in enduring life as well as spiritual development.

7. This is a Sanskrit word which refers to a particular jewel according to Deumar Geshe Tenzin Phuntsok (1725-?). It also means very clear. He has classified three types of *vaidurya* in his book *Dri.Med Shel.Phreng*, which are green, yellow, and white. However, Regent Sangye Gyatso (1653-1705) classifies blue, yellow, and white. Since it has not been identified correctly, I prefer to keep the same name as appears in the text, i.e., *vaidurya*. Different writers have given different names to it and they are: lapis lazuli, beryl, aquamarine, and sapphire.

8. According to the most historical events, Vairotsana, the great translator, paid this homage. He is one of the (seven probationers) first seven monks of Tibet ordained by Acharya Shantaraksita in Samye during the reign of thirty-seventh king Trisong Deutsen (A.D. 718-785) as well as one of the twenty-five disciples of Acharya Padmasambhava. It is also a tradition in Tibet to pay homage in the beginning when translating or writing a book for:

    (a) successful completion of the work,
    (b) to avert the obstacles, and
    (c) to gain merit from working on it.

    Same homage is also seen on the *Yan.Lag brGyad.Pa'i sNying.Po* translated by Great translator Rinchen Sangpo (A.D. 958-1056).

9. They are: excellent resources, excellent physical features, excellent glory, excellent fame, excellent wisdom, and excellent effort.

10. The three mental poisons are: attachment, anger, and delusion.

11. This homage was believed paid by sage *Yid.Las sKyes* (Skt: *Manasija*; Eng: Born from the Mind). Sage *Yid.Las sKyes* was Medicine Buddha's speech emanation, who made request to sage *Rig.Pa'i Ye.Shes* (Skt: *Vidyajnana*; Eng: Wisdom of Awareness) to expound the *gSo.Ba Rig.Pa* (Skt: *Cikitsa Vidya*;

Eng: *Science of Healing*) and was also the collector of this teaching. There is also another notion that sage *Rig.Pa'i Ye.Shes* and sage *Yid.Las sKyes* were actually the Junior Yuthog Yonten Gonpo (A.D. 1126-1202) and his disciple, Sumton Yeshe Zoong, respectively. The proverb by Sumton follows in Tibetan and English:

mKhas.Pa gYu.Thog mGon.Po De
Rig.Pa'i Ye.Shes Lags.Pa 'Dra
Ngos.Rang Yid.Las sKyes.Sam sNyam
Tshe.Rabs Kyi *Bla*.Ma Yin.Par Nges

For me the learned Yuthog Gonpo
Is like *Rig.Pa'i Ye.Shes*
And I consider myself Yid.Las sKyes
He is certainly my guru from previous lives

12. All the teachings Buddha Shakya Muni (625-544 B.C.) gave also embody five excellences. The only difference we see is spoken and heard. In sutra, it reads, "Thus I have heard at one time."

13. Although there are disagreements about identifying *lTa.Na.sDug* among past Tibetan masters, Sangye Gyatso (A.D. 1653-1705) thinks this is Deer Park in Sarnath, Varanasi. To support this, he quotes a verse from *bShad.mDzod Chen.Mo (Treasures of Great Exposition)* which says Buddha Shakya Muni lived "four years in the forest of medicine." He further says the forest of medicine is the abode of sages. Its old names are Rishipatana and Sarangnath. Elder Yuthog Yonten Gonpo (A.D. 708-833) also mentioned that he saw this place as explained in the basis of discourse in his pure vision when he visited India for the third time at the age of thirty-eight. He further says this place lies geographically in the west of Bodh Gaya.

14. The five precious jewels are classified in many ways. Regent Sangye Gyatso, in his commentary book on *rGyud.bZhi*, classifies them as gold, silver, white and red pearl, and *vaidurya*.

15. The Explanatory Tantra's chapter twelve on the Classification of Diseases classifies 404 diseases:

   • 101 disorders are classified according to *Rlung, mKhris.Pa*, and *Bad.Kan*
   • 101 disorders are classified according to principal disorders of single and complex
   • 101 disorders are classified according to site
   • 101 disorders are classified according to type

16. The 1080 types of obstacles are classified as follows:

(a) From delusion arises 360 eunuch or naga and ground spirit which causes *Bad.Kan* disorders.

(b) From attachment arise 360 female demons which cause *Rlung* disorders.

(c) From anger arise 360 male demons which cause *mKhris.Pa* disorders.

17. The examples of hot, sour, and salty tasting medicines are Shing.Kun
(Asafoetida), Da.Trig (Rhus sp.), and Shing.Tsha (cinnamon), respectively.

18. The examples of root, trunk, branch, leaf, flower, and fruit medicines are
Dong.Gra   (Alpinia galanga Willd.), *Thang.Ma sGron.Shing* (Pinus sp.),
A.Za.Mo (Clematis sp.), *Da.Li* (Rhododendron sp.), *lCe.Tsha* (Ranunculus
acris), and *Ka.Ran.Za* (Caesalpinia sepiaria), respectively.

19. Though sandalwood and neem grow in plain and warm areas, they are listed
here because of their cooling power.

20. The examples of bitter, sweet, and astringent tasting medicines are *Tig.Ta*
(Swertia chirata), *Shing.mNgar* (Glycyrrhiza glabra Linn.), and *Li Ga.Dur*
(Berginia ligulata), respectively.

21. The examples of root, trunk, branch, leaf, flower, and fruit medicines are
Bong.dKar (Aconitum heterophyllum Wall), *Tsan.Dan dMar.Po* (Pterocarpus
santalinus), *Ba.Le.Ka* (Aristolochia sp.), *gYa'.Kyi.Ma* (Chrysosplenium sp.),
Na.Ga Ge.Sar (Bombax ceiba), and *rGun.'Brum* (Vitis vinifera L.), respectively.

22. The six vessel organs are stomach, small intestine, large intestine, urinary
bladder, gall bladder, and reproductive organs.

23. The five vital organs are the heart, lungs, liver, spleen, and kidneys.

24. The five kinds of Terminalia chebula are *rNam.rGyal* (Skt: *Vijaya*; Eng:
Victor), *'Jigs.Med* (Skt: *Abaya*; Eng: Fearless), *bDud.rTsi* (Skt: *Amrta*; Eng:
Nectar), *'Phel.Byed* (Increasing), and *sKem.Po* (Dry).

25. Compare this with the following Ayurvedic combinations:

(a)	Earth	+	Water	=	Sweet
(b)	Fire	+	Earth	=	Sour
(c)	Water	+	Fire	=	Salty
(d)	Space	+	Air	=	Bitter
(e)	Fire	+	Air	=	Hot
(f))	Earth	+	Air	=	Astringent

26. *Nyes.Pa gSum* means three afflictions, and it corresponds to the *Tridoshas—*
vata, pitta, kapha—in the Ayurveda, the Indian system of medicine.

27. This refers to blood vessels and the nervous system.

28. The five kinds of calcites are male, female, son, daughter, and neuter calcite.

29. The five kinds of mineral exudates are gold, silver, copper, iron, and lead exudate.

30. This is a chronic hepato-gastrointestinal disease characterized by the simultaneous combination of *Rlung, mKhris.Pa, Bad.Kan,* and blood disorders.

31. *Vaidurya sNgon.Po*—most commentaries refer to this bird as a fabulous creature with wings and bird's feet, but otherwise like a human being. A *Tibetan-English Dictionary* by Rai Sarat Chandra Das refers this to a crane as well as a bird of the height of man that subsists on poisonous drugs. *gYu.Thog dGongs.rGyan, A Medical Dictionary* by Wangdue refers to this as Shang-Shang Te'u, a bird of the size of a peacock with multi-colored feathers. Das also refers Shang-Shang Te'u as a pheasant or a partridge.

32. Buddha Shakya Muni (625-544 BC) manifested himself in the form of Nirmanakaya (Tib: *sPrul.sKu*; Eng: Emanation body) Medicine Buddha.

33. Buddhas are endowed with thirty-two major marks and eighty minor marks.

34. This refers to Terminalia chebula. It is also called myrobalan fruit. See note 24.

35. The two goals or purposes are the purpose of self and the purpose of others.

36. The five wisdoms are mirror-like wisdom, wisdom of discrimination, wisdom of equality, wisdom of accomplishment, and wisdom of reality or absolute.

37. Cause here refers to five poisons: attachment, anger, delusion, pride, and jealousy, and their respective effects are *Rlung, mKhris.Pa, Bad.Kan,* microorganisms, and blood.

38. A god of *gZugs.Khams* (Skt: *rupa dhatu*; Eng: form realm) who conceits himself as creator of all sentient beings and has a resemblance of Brahma.

39. She offered *A.Ru.Ra rNam.rGyal* (Terminalia chebula) to Buddha Shakya Muni when he manifested in the form of a Medicine Buddha.

40. The son of Shiva with six faces who holds a short spear that has a peacock's feather on its tip and rides a peacock. He is also the master of an ancient non-Buddhist sect called Carvaka.

41. Arya Manju Shri, Avalokiteshvara, and Vajra Pani are called the lords of the three families.

42. The personal attendant and cousin of Buddha Shakya Muni who was present at the first Buddhist council sponsored by King Ajatashatru at Rajagrha. He was second in line from the seven hierarchs in succession to Buddha.

43. He was son of King Bimbisara and studied medicine under the son of great sage Atreya. He was crowned thrice the King of Physicians and was the personal physician to Buddha Shakya Muni.

44. The same biography also states eighth day.

45. A chapter on the tradition of Enlightened Master in *gSo.Rig sMan.Gyi Khog.'Bugs*, a medical history by Sangye Gyatso (A.D. 1653-1705), says the Buddha taught *gSo.dPyad 'Bum.Pa (One Hundred Thousand Verses of Healing)* to great god Brahma simultaneous with the second turning of the Wheel of Dharma at *Bya.rGod Phung.po'i Ri* (Vulture's Peak) on the Perfection of Wisdom Sutras. He also taught *gCer.mThong Rig.Pa'i rGyud (The Tantra of Bare Vision)* to the Avalokiteshvara, Brahma, Shariputra, and other

Mahayana disciples at Beta Groves. It also says the latter has 3,500 chapters with 100,000 verses. It is believed that both the former and latter are the same text with two different names. If that is true, then the teaching gods received should be translated as *One Hundred Thousand Verses of Healing* and not the *Healing Therapy Vase*. The *rGyud.bZhi* and all the other related works read '*Bum.Pa* and not *Bum.Pa*. The former '*Bum* means 100,000 and *pa* means to possess. The latter *Bum.Pa* means vase. Hence the teachings they heard are:

(a) The gods heard *gSo.dPyad 'Bum.Pa* (*One Hundred Thousand Verses of Healing*)

(b) The sages heard *Tsa.Ra.Ka sDe.brGyad* (*Charaka Ashtanga*)

(c) The non-Buddhists heard *dBang.Phyug Nag.Po'i rGyud* (*Tantra of Black Ishvara*)

(d) The Buddhists heard *Rigs.gSum mGon.Po'i sKor* (*the teachings pertaining to the Lord of the Three Families*)

46. This refers to sage *Yid.Las sKyes* (Skt: Manasija; Eng: Born from the Mind).

Chapter Two

1. This is also a synonym for Terminalia chebula.

2. The ten directions are the four cardinal directions, the four sub-directions, zenith, and nadir.

3. The three mental non-virtuous actions are covetousness, malicious intent, and wrong view.

4. Sentient beings are of six types, and they are gods, human beings, demigods, hell beings, hungry ghosts, and animals.

5. The second of the five Buddha families (Skt: *dhyani*; Tib: *Rigs*). His abode (paradise) is *mNgon.Par dGa'.Ba* (Skt: *Abhinandan*; Eng: Manifesting Joy) and is in the East. His other names are Mi.'Khrugs.Pa (Skt: Akshobya) and rDo.rJe Sems.dPa' (Skt: Vajrasattva).

6. Receiving teachings, wealth, wishes (free from sickness, long life, happiness, and respect, etc.), and liberation are called four worldly excellences.

7. Four verbal non-virtuous actions are lying, slander, harsh speech, and idle gossip.

8. The fourth of the five Buddha families. His abode is *bDe.Ba Can* (Skt: *Sukhavati*; Eng: Land of Bliss or Great Bliss) and is in the West. His other names are *Tshe.dPag Med* (*Amitayus*) and '*Od.dPag Med* (*Amitabha*). They are designated according to the form of existence or body.

9. This indicates no fear, no timidity, and no hesitation in asking about teachings.

10. A group of ten different forms of medicine, such as decoction, powders, etc., is called pacification medicine. Their action is to balance the imbalances in its respective site.

11. A group of medicines of purgatives and emetics, etc., is called cleansing med-

icines. Their action is to cause the arisal of disorder and then to expel it from the lower (anal canal) or above (mouth) doors.

12. Venesection and moxibustions, therapy, which removes disease from outside of body and pacifies it, are called accessory therapy. Compress therapy, medicinal bath, and massage come into the category of smooth accessory therapy. Venesection, moxibustions, and spoon surgery come into the category of coarse accessory therapy.

13. They are: (1) easy to cure, (2) difficult to cure, (3) scarcely treatable, and (4) to be abstained from treating.

14. This refers to 'Or, the edema of the skin vesicles.

15. This refers to dMu.Chu, the edema of the internal organs.

16. This is also called a junction of fever between melting and freezing. This explains differentiating between hot and cold disorders.

17. This refers to the initial stage fever. Owing to the association of Bad.Kan and Rlung, the fever is prevented from manifesting fully and the resultant symptoms are: uneven physical warmth with rise of flesh fever (surface fever; Sha.Drod Che.Ba) during the dusk, frequent yawning, lethargy, bitter taste in mouth, headache, pain in the calves and joints, shivering that attracts the sun and fire, nightmares, and great mental stress.

18. This refers to a fever, which is associated with the Rlung. As fever declines with the remedies, the Rlung rises, and the Rlung fan the remnants of the fever. Empty fever is like the remnants of fire in the blacksmith's hearth (fireplace). Though Rlung is cold, as long as it fans the fever will continue to rise and will not stop until the Rlung stops fanning it. It is also like an empty sac which has been distended by air.

19. Though externally it shows symptoms of cold, in reality, the fever is hidden internally under the cover of Bad.Kan and Rlung. It is like a fire under the cover of ash.

20. This refers to a fever, which has become complicated due to the combination of Rlung, blood, and lymph.

21. This fever ensues after a fall, accident, injury, beating, or being trapped under a collapsed building or landslide. All of these cause the bodily constituents to scatter, disturb blood, and raise the heat of mKhris.Pa.

22. This refers to a fever which burns the bodily constituents. mKhris.Pa, being hot when disturbed, raises warmth in blood, strikes lungs, liver, and many other organs, and is painful and expectorates blood-stained phlegm or blood and phlegm.

23. This includes diabetes also.

24. This includes burns, food choking, and frostbite.

25. This ensues due to spreading or scattering and disturbances of the Nyes.Pa. This in turn causes the unripening of the nutritional essence and proliferates the bad (waste) blood. Bad blood then diffuses in the channels; Rlung rolls it and then solidifies it.

26. *Surya* is a Sanskirt word that means sun. This refers to a disease that ensues after the proliferation of bad (waste and dead) blood and lymph in the vessels of vital and vessel organs causing swelling, pain, and finally pus formation.

27. There are six types of swelling of the testicles. They are caused mainly by the disturbances of the descending *Rlung,* including inguinal hernia. Strain on inguinal canal by descending *Rlung* disturbances causes protrusion of the intestine, etc., into the scrotum and is associated with swelling and hanging of one side or both.

28. This is a lymph, blood, and *Bad.Kan* combined disorder characterized by mild pain and swelling of the legs.

29. This refers to a fresh menstrual blood disorder and *Rlung* combined chronic menstrual blood disorder.

30. This refers to a specific and acute menstrual blood disorder and uterine tumors, etc., twenty-seven types of disorders.

31. This refers to pregnancy related symptoms and the problems associated with delivery, etc., eight types of disorders.

32. This refers to a demonic effect that penetrates a person's body, speech, and mind and then takes over his/her actions. There are eighteen types of elemental spirits.

33. This is a mental disorder that ensues due to diversion of mental consciousness in the heart's channel by disturbances of *Nyes.Pa*, grief, poison, and insane causing spirits in association with king spirit.

34. This refers to a mental disorder which ensues due to disturbances of *Nyes.Pa*, poison, and amnesia causing spirits in association with planetary spirits. Organs involved are heart and brain.

35. This refers to a stroke. An associate spirit is *Naga*.

36. This refers to leprosy, etc., thirty-six types of skin diseases caused by the ripening of past bad karma in conjunction with *Naga* and black (blood and *mKhris.Pa* combined) lymph disorder.

37. This refers to plants and animals bearing poisons.

38. The decoctions mature fevers, withdraw disorders that have spread throughout the body, and separate diseased and healthy blood. They are prescribed first because of their sharp and quick actions which are due to the functional effects of taste.

39. The powders are prescribed when decoction fails to pacify a disorder. Owing to their post-digestive functional effects, their action is slower than the decoctions.

40. The pills are prescribed in the end to uproot the disorder. The effect of pills ensue after complete digestion and their action is slower than the above two medicines. The longer the medicines take to show their effects on disease, the better they are at pacifying the disease from the root.

41. Though decoctions, powders, and pills pacify most disorders, pastes are

expounded for the elimination of chronic disorders affected to the channels (blood vessels and nerves), joints, and skin.

42. Medicinal butters are prescribed after all other treatments to rejuvenate and strengthen one's bodily constituents and vitality and to promote the functions of all the organs and the clarity of the five senses, organs, and mind.

43. They are prescribed to eliminate the cold disorders caused mainly by *Bad.Kan* imbalances.

44. They are prescribed to eliminate most of the hot disorders.

45. They are prescribed to eliminate most of the disorders associated with *Rlung*.

46. The jewel medicines are two times more powerful than all other medicines and often prescribed as a last resort to pacify very chronic, serious, and deeply buried diseases.

47. The herbal compounds are expounded to counteract immediate disorders. Since herbs grow everywhere, if one is knowledgeable about the benefits of herbs growing in the surrounding areas, one can utilize those as a countermeasure against immediate disorders.

48. This is done to prevent *Rlung* imbalances as well as adverse effects of the purgatives, etc., cleansing works.

49. They are recommended to pacify diseases above the neck base, including the head and sense organs. Nasal medications are of two kinds, peaceful and drastic.

50. This refers to drastic countermeasures to evacuate small and large intestine diseases from the downward (anal canal).

51. This is the most powerful cleansing therapy, which is recommended to evacuate the chronic and stubborn blood and *mKhris.Pa* disorder and other poisoning diseases through the urinary tract system.

52. This is recommended for dual and tri-*Nyes.Pa* combined predominant *mKhris.Pa* imbalances and particularly against rigidity and stiffening of the channels (blood vessels and nerves), tendons, and ligaments.

53. This is recommended to pacify dual and tri-*Nyes.Pa* combined predominant *Rlung* disorder.

54. This is recommended as a last resort when all other treatments fail.

Chapter Three

1. *Lags* is an honorific word which is added after a person's name to show respect.

2. This refers to sage *Yid.Las sKyes* and four groups of disciples.

3. The roots and trunks, etc., are explained in great detail in the same (third) chapter and in the fourth and fifth chapters of the Root Tantra. The origin of metaphor to tantras and chapters are rooted in the Elder Yuthog Yonten Gonpo's biography.

4. The Tibetan term for humor is *Nad* (disease) and *Nyes.Pa* (Skt: *dosha*; Eng:

affliction). *Nyes.Pa* refers to the body's energies, the *Rlung*, *mKhris.Pa*, and *Bad.Kan*. Although their function is to sustain and support life, they also have the potential to cause affliction. When disturbed, they cause abnormal functioning of the seven bodily constituents and the three excretions, resulting in physical and mental suffering. They are therefore called Nad or *Nyes.Pa*.

5. In *Rin.Chen Phreng.Ba (Jewel Rosary)*, Chagpa had mentioned that this *Rlung* resides in the spinal cord and particularly in the brain. See *gYu.Thog dGongs.rGyan*, the *Tibetan Medical Dictionary* by Wangdue.

6. Arya Nagarjuna, in his book called *Zla.Ba'i rGyal.Po (King of Moon)*, says this *Rlung* resides in the lungs.

7. *Pho.Ba* has two meanings, the stomach and to move. Here it refers to the latter and hence, the whole alimentary canal should be understood as *Pho.Ba*. However, it refers specifically to the large intestine and this is most likely an ascending colon.

8. It refers to seven bodily constituents and three excretions. They are called objects of harming because these are the objects on which the three *Nyes.Pa* function. Imbalance in *Nyes.Pa* causes malfunctioning of the ten objects.

9. Though the Tibetan term *gZhang* refers to the anal canal, my assumption is it implies to the sacral region. This is based on my understanding from reading and studying the functions of the nervous system as wells as its anatomy.

10. The digested and undigested part of *Pho.Ba* refers to the large intestine and stomach, respectively. Between them lies the small intestine. See note 7 for a description of *Pho.Ba*.

11. It is also called the red transformer because of its action.

12. In *rGyud.bzhi*, the location of supporting *Bad.Kan* has not been pin pointed or mentioned clearly. Therefore, I think this refers indirectly to either the heart or lungs. The thirteenth chapter, from an *Oral Instruction's Tantra of rGyud.b2hi*, a chapter on the *clearing the basis of errors on contraindications of hot and cold disorders* says the heart is a base of *Rlung* and *Bad.Kan*. Therefore, when fever diffuses into the heart, the symptoms resemble those of the cold (*Bad.Kan*) *Rlung* disorder. The other point is the thirty-fifth chapter from an *Oral Instruction's Tantra of rGyud.bzhi*, a chapter on healing of lungs diseases says, in general, a *Bad.Kan* is located in the lungs. Therefore, a patient with lungs disease feels better during the summer and worse during the winter. Similarly, a patient feels better during the day and worse during the night.

13. This refers to the stomach.

14. It is also called *brTas.Byed* (empowering *Bad.Kan*).

15. This refers to the brain.

16. They are faith, moral discipline, generosity, hearing, sense of shame, dread of blame, and wisdom.

17. *Ma.Rig.Pa* is one of the six root delusions as well as first in line of the twelve links of dependent origination. The *Wheel of Life* uses the symbol of an old

blind woman with a cane in her hand for support.

18. This refers to blood vessels.

19. This indirectly reveals the perverse winter season.

20. This refers to the general entrance of the diseases in relation to their corresponding passages. It does not imply that every disease follows the sequence as described since there are diseases of contrary sequence as well. The skin and muscles, and vessels and bones, and *Don.lNga* and *sNod.Drug*, in turn, represent external, middle, and internal body.

21. These are the sites where imbalanced *Nyes.Pa* reveals their sign and symptoms.

22. The chapter on actions and classifications of the body of Explanatory Tantra delineates the life-stage limit as: childhood, from birth to sixteen years of age; adulthood, from seventeen to seventy years of age; and old age, from the age of seventy-one onwards.

23. All of these diseases occurred under the influence of past (negative) karma.

24. The chapter on signs of death of explanatory Tantra says, loss of one's outer, inner, and life (vessel) constituents, namely muscles (function), food (intake), and channels (blood vessels and nerves) (function) indicate certain death. His Holiness the XIVth Dalai Lama explains different conditions of dying through *In Kindness, Clarity, and Insight*. They are: to die when one's life span has been exhausted; another, to die when one's merit has been exhausted; and the third is to die unexpectedly, as in a car accident.

25. They are diet, behavioral patterns, medicines, and accessory therapy.

26. *Bla* (vital life force) is said to be the mother of life. Like a mother, *Bla* sustain one's life.

27. The chapter on specific healing techniques of explanatory Tantra specifically mentions this as a resultant of excessive or perverse intake of food and medicines possessing the following flavors:

Rlung disorder:	Excessively salty tasting food and medicine pacifies *Rlung* but increases *mKhris.Pa* disorders.
Rlung disorder:	Excessively sweet tasting food and medicine pacifies *Rlung* but increases *Bad.Kan* disorders.
Rlung disorder:	By ingesting hot tasting food and medicine, *Rlung* is not pacified, which increases *mKhris.Pa* disorders.
Rlung disorder:	By ingesting bitter tasting food and medicine, *Rlung* is not pacified, which increases *Bad.Kan* disorders.
mKhris.Pa disorder:	Excessively bitter tasting food and medicine pacifies *mKhris.Pa* but increases *Rlung* disorders.
mKhris.Pa disorder:	Excessively sweet tasting food and medicine pacifies *mKhris.Pa* but increases *Bad.Kan* disorders.
mKhris.Pa disorder:	By ingesting hot tasting food and medicine,

156

	mKhris.Pa is not pacified, which increases *Rlung* disorders.
mKhris.Pa disorder:	By ingesting salty tasting food and medicine, *mKhris.Pa* is not pacified, which increases *Bad.Kan* disorders.
Bad.Kan disorder:	Excessively hot tasting food and medicine pacifies *Bad.Kan* but increases *Rlung* disorders.
Bad.Kan disorder:	Excessively sour tasting food and medicine pacifies *Bad.Kan* but increases *mKhris.Pa* disorders.
Bad.Kan disorder:	By ingesting bitter tasting food and medicine, *Bad.Kan* is not pacified, which increases *Rlung* disorders.
Bad.Kan disorder:	By ingesting salty tasting food and medicine, *Bad.Kan* is not pacified, which increases *mKhris.Pa* disorders.

Chapter Five

1. Leaves marked with an asterisk represent substances that are in the text which in actuality do help alleviate *Rlung* disorder but are not practiced by Tibetans in their daily lives.

2. Though *Sha.Chen* (great meat) refers to human flesh (a meat of a healthy person who died suddenly), *Sha.lNga* (five meats) in addition refers to the meat of an elephant, a horse, a dog, a peacock, or beef.

3. *Zan.Chang* is prepared from *rTsam.Pa* (roasted barley flour), the staple diet of Tibet.

4. The text lists curd and buttermilk under food.

5. *mDzo.Mo* itself is a cross-bred offspring of a yak with a cow or an ox with a *'Bri* (female yak).

6. Tibetan tea is made from boiling tea leaves in the water. It is then poured in the churn and added to the butter, milk, and salt and churned again and again until they mix well. It is then strained and served for a drink.

7. This is named after a legend, which says: *gNod.sByin rGod.Ma Kha* is a very huge fire of constantly burning coal or formation of crystal fire, which looks like a mouth of a mare. It lies very deep in the ocean and is a thousand times hotter than ordinary fire. Because of that, it is believed that though all the waters on earth ultimately go down to the ocean, it is never spilled over as the fire dries them. Similarly, this medicinal compound contains all cold disorders however powerful they may be.

   The other legend says: In ancient time, a son with a face of a mare was born to a *yaksha* (harmful spirit) who had a very strong digestive power and so whatever food he eats digests with ease and similarly it enables one to digest whatever one eats by promoting the power of the digestive heat. The digestive heat here refers to a concept similar to the "Triple heaters" in

Chinese medicine or the *Tri Agni* in Ayurveda. In Tibetan medicine, the three digestive heats are Decomposing *Bad.Kan*, Digestive *mKhris.Pa*, and Fire accompanying *Rlung*.

Diagnosis by Pulse Examination:
1. The left channel in our body, which is white in color, stands adjacent to the central energy channel. It runs from the level of the eyebrows to the point between the eyebrow and the navel and represents the method aspect of the path. The specific details vary according to the lineage of the practice concerned.
2. The right channel in our body, which is red in color, stands adjacent to the central energy channel. It runs from the level of the eyebrows to the point between the eyebrow and the navel and represents the wisdom aspect of the path. The specific details vary according to the lineage of the practice concerned.
3. The central channel in our body is straight, hollow, luminous, and blue and runs from the top of the head beneath the soft spot on the skull called the "Gate of Brahma," to a space located four finger widths beneath the navel. It represents the absolute aspect, consciousness, and non-dual wisdom.
4. This refers to cardiovascular disorders, including hypertension.
5. This is a chronic *mKhris.Pa* and blood prominent hepato-gastrointestinal disorder characterized by the simultaneous combination of *Rlung* and *Bad.Kan*.
6. This refers to the *Rlung* and *Bad.Kan* combined lymph disorder.
7. This refers to *Bad.Kan* caused indigestion which ensues pale complexion.
8. This refers to the *Rlung* and *Bad.Kan* caused benign tumor. It appears mostly in the stomach and large intestine.
9. This refers to an acute lung infection.
10. One can apply this knowledge to an injury to other parts of the body.
11. This was from *gSo.Rig rGyud.bZhi'i Grel.Chen Drang.Srong Zhal.Lung* by Thoru Tsenam. In *Vaidurya sNgon.Po* and other commentary books, they say the pulse beats fast and trembles like *Nya.Mo rNgams'Dra*. That means when a life of a fish is threatened by taking off from a water, the fish trembles and tries to run from the person's hand. When he holds lightly the fish tries to leap and when he presses strongly, there is no movement.
12. Following surgery for the removal of the spleen or the right or left kidney, one may also miss the pulse beat of the respective organ, but that does not represent the death pulse.
13. According to Dr. Lobsang Tenzin Rinpoche, one should also know how to interpret the person's life span by weeks, months, and years on the basis of patient's physical condition, i.e., very serious, serious, and not serious.
14. This is an instruction given by Elder Yuthog Yonten Gonpo (A.D. 708-833) to his disciple.

Diagnosis by Urine Examination

1. Intense hunger and fasting, listed under section 1. Prerequisite Conditions of Diagnosis by Pulse Examination, are interpreted as to avoid a mistaken diagnosis of a cold disorder due to a low and weak pulse beat. But here, fasting or lack of food is interpreted as to avoid false characteristics of *Rlung* disorder. The former interprets in general and the latter as more specifically. In general, both of them belong to the same category. See Branch 9: Summation of Part One: Chapter Three: The Basis of Normal and Abnormal Body.

2. *Bad.Kan* and *mKhris.Pa* are by nature the two opposing energies of our body. *Bad.Kan* represents the cold and *mKhris.Pa* the hot. When these two energies become out of balance, each tries to overcome the other and the conflict starts.

3. This is a blood and *mKhris.Pa* combined lymph disorder.

4. The disturbances in the *Rlung* fan the poisoning, *Bad.Kan sMug.Po*, or chronic fever and spreads throughout the body.

5. This information is taken from the *rGyud.bZhi'i rNam.bShad* by Kyempa Tsewang. *rGyud.bZhi* and other commentary books on it (*rGyud.bZhi*) explain *sPu.rtse Dra.Ba*, which means "like the tip of a hair strand."

6. The fever spreads throughout the body due to *Rlung* disturbances.

7. This refers to a cooling power that all four remedies have in common such as diet, behavior, medicine, and the accessory therapy.

8. This refers to a warming power that all four remedies have in common such as diet, behavior, medicine, and the accessory therapy.

9. That reflects *rGyud.bZhi*, the main medical text. A commentary book on *rGyud.bZhi*, called *Vaidurya sNgon.Po* by Desi Sangye Gyatso, also reflects about an appearance of a suture-like line from sediments or scum in a particular grid when the urine is still and not stirred.

10. This can be understood from a patient's worsening condition whenever the (same) person is visiting him/her. The intention of this person may be good, but the spirit accompanying this person is believed to be behind the patient's worsening condition.

11. *Nagas* or serpent spirits abide in fountains, rivers, lakes, and subterranean realms. They are regarded as belonging to the animal class and are also believed to be the guardian of great treasures underground. They have control over rain, ponds, rivers, and soil productivity. Some are helpers while others can bring retribution if disturbed. Often, in Buddhist art and in written accounts, they are portrayed as being half man and half snake. Generally serpents and snakes are recognized as *nagas*.

12. This is a space-dwelling spirit found in rivers, lakes, trees, rocks, and ruins of sacred sites.

13. *Sa.bDag* means lord of earth or owner of the Earth. This is a ground-dwelling spirit having influence at the locality or sites.

1. This is an instruction given by Elder Yuthog Yonten Gonpo (A.D. 708-833) to his disciple.

Secondary Diagnosis

1. In *bDud.rTsi'i Chu.rGyun* (Stream of Nectar's Water), a commentary on the Explanatory Tantra by Jangpa Namgyal Daksang mentions the sweet, sour, and salty tastes.
2. *Vaidurya sNgon.Po*, a commentary on *rGyud.bZhi* by Desi Sangye Gyastso, does not explain how the nature of the person resembles a vulture, fox, etc. The resemblance of a person's nature to animals is added here from *bDud.rTsi'i Chu.rGyun* (Stream of Nectar's Water), a commentary on the Explanatory Tantra by Jangpa Namgyal Dagsang (A.D. 1295-1376).
3. This results due to improper maturation of nutritional essences into blood by the complexion transforming *mKhris.Pa* in the liver. Proliferation of such unripe blood is called bad blood.
4. This is an infant's liver disorder in which it is believed that the liver of the child slips out of its original site. This is perhaps an enlargement of the child's liver.
5. The diffusion of *Rlung* and *Bad.Kan* combined cold disorder in the digestive *mKhris.Pa* site spreads bile in the channels and the symptoms associated are: low body temperature, indigestion, yellowish sclera, urine and body, slow pulse rate, and particularly the pale stool.

REFERENCES

1. Yuthog, Yonten Gonpo (Younger). *bDud.rTsi sNying.Po Yan.Lag brGyad.Pa gSang.Ba Man.Ngag gi rGyud*. Lhasa: Chakpori Press, 1888.

2. Yuthog, Yonten Gonpo (Younger). *sMan.gZhung Cha. Lag bCo.brGyad*. Men-Tsee-Khang: Dharamsala, 1999.

3. Gyatso, Desi Sangye. *gSo.Ba Rig.Pa'i bsTan.bCos sMan.Bla'i dGongs.rGyan rGyud.bZhi'i gSal.Byed Vaidurya sNgon.Po'i Ma.lli.ka Zhes Bya.Ba bZhugs.So*. Lhasa: Zhol Press, 1893.

4. Zurkhar, Lodoe Gyalpo. *rGyud.bZhi'i 'Grel.Pa Mes.Po'i Zhal.Lung*. Lhasa: Zhol Press, 1893.

5. Norbu, Khyenrab. *rTsa.rGyud sDong.'Grems gSo.Rig rGya.mTsho'i sNying.Po*. Sarnath: Tibetan Monastery Press, 1966.

6. Tsenam, Thoru. *gSo.Rig rGyud.bZhi'i 'Grel.Chen Drang.Srong Zhal.Lung*, Vol. 1. Zi.Khron Mi.Rigs dPe.sKrun Khang, 2001.

7. Tsenam, Thoru. *gSo.Rig rGyud.bZhi'i 'Grel.Chen Drang.Srong Zhal.Lung*, Vol. 4. Zi.Khron Mi.Rigs dPe.sKrun Khang, 2001.

8. Tsenam, Thoru. *gSo.rig rGyud.bZhi'i 'Grel.Chen Drang.Srong Zhal.lung*, Vol. 5. Zi.Khron Mi.Rigs dPe. sKrun Khang, 2001.

9. Gyatso, Desi Sangye. *Man.Ngag Lhan.Thabs*. mTsho.sNgon Mi.Rigs dPe.sKrun Khang, 1991.

10. Me.Lha, Sangye. *sNyan.brGyud Be.Bum Nag.Po*. Publishers unknown.

11. Kongtrul, Yonten Gyatso. *gSo.rig Zin.Tig gCes.bsDus*. mTsho.sNgon Mi.dMangs dPe.sKrun Khang, 1976.

12. Dorje, Zurkhar Nyamnyi. *Man.Ngag Bye.Ba Ring. bSrel.* Kansu Mi.Rigs dPe.sKrun Khang, 1993.

13. Wangdue. *gSo.Ba Rig.Pa'i Tshig.mDzod gYu.Thog dGongs.rGyan.* Mi.Rigs dPe.sKrun Khang, 1982.

14. Deumar, Tenzin Phuntsok. *sMan.Gyi Nus.Pa Dri.Med Shel.Phreng.* Dharamsala: 1994.

15. Karma, Choephel. *bDud.rTsi sMan.Gyi 'Khrung.dPe Legs.bShad Nor.Bu'i Phreng.mDzes.* Tibet: 1993.

16. Tendar, Sogpo Lungrig. *rGyud.bZhi'i brDa.bKrol rNam.rGyal A.Ru.Ra'i Phreng.Ba'i mDzes.rGyan.* Mi.Rigs dPe.sKrun Khang, 1986.

17. Tashi, Jowo Lhundup and Choedrak, Darmo Menrampa Lobsang. *gYu.Thog gSar.rNying Gi rNam.Thar.* Mi.Rigs dPe.sKrun Khang, 1982.

18. Gyatso, Desi Sangye. *gSo.Rig sMan.Gyi Khog.'Bugs.* Kansu Mi.Rigs dPe.sKrun Khang, Kansu, Tibet: 1982.

19. Dawa, Menrampa. *Bod.Kyi gSo.Rig sMan.Ris gSal. Ba'i Me.Long.* Dharamsala: Tibetan Medical and Astro Institute, 1993.

20. Dorjee, Menrampa Gawa. *'Khrung.dPe Dri.Med Shel.Gyi Me.Long.* Mi.Rigs dPe.sKrun Khang, 1995.

21. *Bod.lJongs rGyun.sPyod Krung.dByi'i sMan.Rigs.* Bod. lJong Mi.dMangs dPe.sKrun Khang, 1973.

22. *gSo.Rig rGyud.bZhi'i sDong.'Grems 'Dod.'Byung Nor.Bu'i mDzod.* Mi.Rigs dPe.sKrun Khang, 1988.

23. Dawa. *Bod.Kyi gSo.Ba Rig.Pa Las sMan.rDzas sByor. bZo'i Lag.Len gSang.sGo 'Byed.Pa'i lDe.Mig.* New Delhi, Ri Drag Publication: 2003.

24. Phakhol. *Yan.Lag brGyad.Pa'i sNying.Po bsDus.Pa.* Mi.Rigs dPe.sKrun Khang, 1989.

25. mNgon.dGa', Dawa. *sMan.dPyad Yan.Lag brGyad.Pa'i sNying.Po'i rNam.Par 'Grel.Pa'i Tshig.Gi Don.Gyi Zla.Zer Zhes Bya.Ba bZhugs.So.* Mi.Rigs dPe.sKrun Khang, 1992.

26. *Bod.Kyi gSo.Rig Slob.Deb*, Vol. 1. Men-Tsee-Khang, Dharamsala, 1997.

27. *Bod.Kyi gSo.Rig Slob.Deb*, Vol. 2. Men-Tsee-Khang, Dharamsala, 1997.

28. *sMan.dPyad Zla.Ba'i rGyal.Po*. Men-Tsee-Khang, Dharamsala

29. Deumar, Tenzin Phuntsok. *gSo.Rig gCes.bTus Rin.Chen Phreng.Ba*. mTsho.sNgon Mi.Rigs dPe.sKrun Khang, 1993.

30. Dagsang, Jangpa Namgyal. bShad.Pa'i rGyud.Kyi rGya.Cher Grel.Ba bDud.rTsi'i Chu.rGyun Zhes Bya.Ba bZhugs.So.Mi.Rigs dPe.sKrun Khang, 2002.

31. Tsona, Lobsang Tsultrim and Dakpa, Tenzing. *Fundamentals of Tibetan Medicine*. Men-Tsee-Khang: Dharamsala, 2001.

32. Paljor, Thokmay and Dakpa, Tenzing. *Guide to the Exhibition on Tibetan Medicine & Astrology*. Men-Tsee-Khang: Dharamsala, 1995.

33. Clifford, Terry. *Tibetan Buddhist Medicine & Psychiatry, The Diamond Healing*. Delhi, Motilal Banarsidass Publishers: 1994.

34. Dhonden, Yeshi. *Health Through Balance*. New York, Snow Lion Publications: 1986.

35. Dhonden, Yeshi. *Healing From The Source*. New York, Snow Lion Publication: 2000.

36. Clark, Barry. *The Quintessence Tantras of Tibetan Medicine*. New York, Snow Lion Publications: 1995.

37. Bakhru, H. K. *Herbs That Heal*. Delhi, Orient Paperbacks: 1995.

38. Rigzin, Tsepak. *Tibetan-English Dictionary of Buddhist Terminology*. Dharamsala, Library of Tibetan Works and Archives: 1986.

39. Das, Rai Sarat Chandra. *A Tibetan English Dictionary*. Delhi, Motilal Banarsidass: 1902.

40. *Bod-rGya Tshig-mDzod Chen-Mo*. Mi-Rigs dPe-sKrun Khang, 1993.

41. Sam.Bod sKad.gNyis Shan.sByar gSer.Gyi Phreng.mDzes. Kansu Mi.Rigs. dPe.Skrun Khang, 1996.

42. *Complete Home Medical Guide*. New York, Crown Publishers, Inc: 1985.

43. *Human Body*. New York, Dorling Kindersley Publishing, Inc.: 2001.

44. Werner, David. *Where There Is No Doctor*. Palo Alto, The Hesperian Foundation: 1977.

45. *Webster's New World Dictionary*. New York: Simon and Schuster, Inc., 1987.